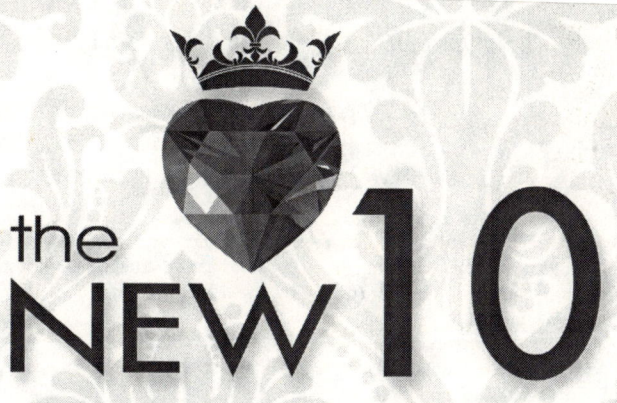

the NEW 10
REDEFINING BEAUTY

40 Days to Creating a
Boldly Beautiful Life From the Inside Out

DAWN MCINTYRE

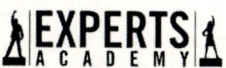

an imprint of Morgan James Publishing
NEW YORK

the NEW 10
REDEFINING BEAUTY

40 Days to Creating a
Boldly Beautiful Life From the Inside Out

by DAWN MCINTYRE

© 2010 Dawn McIntyre. All rights reserved.

No part of this publication may be reproduced or transmitted in any form or by any means, mechanical or electronic, including photocopying and recording, or by any information storage and retrieval system, without permission in writing from author or publisher (except by a reviewer, who may quote brief passages and/or show brief video clips in a review).

Disclaimer: The Publisher and the Author make no representations or warranties with respect to the accuracy or completeness of the contents of this work and specifically disclaim all warranties, including without limitation warranties of fitness for a particular purpose. No warranty may be created or extended by sales or promotional materials. The advice and strategies contained herein may not be suitable for every situation. This work is sold with the understanding that the Publisher is not engaged in rendering legal, accounting, or other professional services. If professional assistance is required, the services of a competent professional person should be sought. Neither the Publisher nor the Author shall be liable for damages arising herefrom. The fact that an organization or website is referred to in this work as a citation and/or a potential source of further information does not mean that the Author or the Publisher endorses the information the organization or website may provide or recommendations it may make. Further, readers should be aware that internet websites listed in this work may have changed or disappeared between when this work was written and when it is read.

ISBN 978-1-60037-757-0 (paperback)

Published by:

EXPERTS ACADEMY PRESS
an imprint of
Morgan James Publishing
1225 Franklin Ave. Ste 325
Garden City, NY 11530-1693
Toll Free 800-485-4943
www.MorganJamesPublishing.com

Interior Design by:
Bonnie Bushman
bbushman@bresnan.net

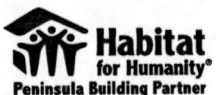

In an effort to support local communities, raise awareness and funds, Morgan James Publishing donates one percent of all book sales for the life of each book to Habitat for Humanity.
Get involved today, visit
www.HelpHabitatForHumanity.org.

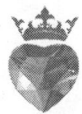

ACKNOWLEDGMENTS

I would like to express my deepest love and gratitude to my daughter, Kennedy. Her unwavering faith in me during many turbulent times was truly my inspiration to grow and heal to become a beautiful woman and an example of who she is by the very nature of her being.

I dedicate this book to you, Kennedy (angel face).

I would also like to thank my sister, Cheryl, for your love, support, and constant encouragement. You never let me give up, even under the toughest of circumstances.

I would also like to thank all of my ex-husbands. You know who you are ☺; you helped me to face my deepest fears and darkest shadows and to embrace the beauty of me, wholly and completely, as a result. You were my greatest teachers.

Finally, I would like to thank my friends. Your support has not gone unnoticed: Ruth Alexander, Michaela Hutchison, Kari Dunlop, Graham Stone, Dwayne Klassen, Sarah Straub, Dale Schnell, Cory Royal, Paul and Melanie Lackan and Rod and Kelly Martin.

All my love,
Dawn

CONTENTS

Acknowledgments iii
Introduction: vii
The New 10 Beauty Quotient Quiz xiii

MY THOUGHTS ARE UGLY. MY THOUGHTS ARE BEAUTIFUL. 1

Day 1:   I Hide from My Fears. I Face My Fears. 3
Day 2:   Who Cares What I Think? I Care What I Think. 7
Day 3:   My Mind Is Closed. My Mind Is Open. 11
Day 4:   Failure Will Destroy Me. Failure Makes Me Stronger. 15
Day 5:   Anger Is Bad. Anger Is Healthy. 19
Day 6:   I Always Worry. I Never Worry. 23
Day 7:   If I'm Rejected, I'll Die! If I'm Rejected, I Will Survive. 27
Day 8:   I Am Worthless. I Am Priceless. 31
Day 9:   I Like to Feel Safe. I Like to Feel Challenged. 35
Day 10: The World Is My Enemy. The World Is My Friend. 39

I HATE MY BODY. I LOVE MY BODY. 43

Day 11: I Give My Body What I Want. I Give My Body
           What It Needs. 45
Day 12: I Am Weak and Sick. I Am Healthy and Strong. 49
Day 13: I Sit Down and Vegetate. I Get Up and Dance! 53
Day 14: I Don't Have Time to Breathe! I Make Time to Breathe. ... 57
Day 15: I Don't Need Vitamins. I Need Vitamins, Minerals,
           and Antioxidants. 61

Day 16:	My Core Is Weak. My Core Is Strong.	65
Day 17:	I Hide from My Sexuality. I Embrace My Sexuality.	69
Day 18:	I Am a Mess. I Am Perfect.	73
Day 19:	I Hide My Body. I Flaunt My Body.	77
Day 20	I Have an Ugly Smile. I Have a Beautiful Smile.	81

I IGNORE MY SPIRIT. I EMBRACE MY SPIRIT. ... 85

Day 21:	I Fear the Universe. I Trust the Universe.	87
Day 22:	I Have a Soul? I Have a Soul!	91
Day 23:	I Am Powerless. I Am Powerful.	95
Day 24:	I Follow the Herd. I Lead by Example.	99
Day 25:	I Have Nothing to Be Grateful For. I Have Everything to Be Grateful For.	103
Day 26:	I Ignore My Heart. I Listen to My Heart.	107
Day 27:	I Have No Imagination. I Use My Imagination.	111
Day 28:	I Don't Want Much. I Want It All!	115
Day 29:	I Cheat Myself. I Treat Myself.	119
Day 30:	Life Is a Tragedy. Life Is a Comedy.	123

MY LIFE IS ORDINARY. MY LIFE IS EXTRAORDINARY. ... 127

Day 31:	I Am Unconscious. I Am Conscious.	129
Day 32:	I Am a Doer. I Am a Be-er.	133
Day 33:	I Live in the Past. I Live in the Now.	137
Day 34:	I Don't Want to Grow Old. I Can't Wait to Grow Old.	141
Day 35:	When Things Go Wrong, I Go Crazy! When Things Go Wrong, I Am Calm.	145
Day 36:	Just Say No. Just Say YES!	149
Day 37:	I Hide My Dark Side. I Embrace My Dark Side.	153
Day 38:	I Deserve Nothing. I Deserve Everything!	157
Day 39:	I Make Things Happen. I Let Things Happen.	161
Day 40:	I Am Impatient. I Am Patient.	165

Conclusion 169

The New 10 Beauty Quotient Quiz 171

Introduction:

Meet the New 10

I remember the first time I heard a woman referred to as a "10."

I was just entering my teens when the movie the term originated from was released. Bo Derek co-starred in the 1979 Blake Edwards film *10* with Dudley Moore. Dudley Moore was torn between his love for another woman, played by Julie Andrews, and his obsession with Bo Derek. The movie created instant stardom for Bo Derek and she became an overnight sex symbol.

Suddenly the world had an "official" standard for beauty. It included being tall and blonde, and having a golden tan, a killer smile, and a body that looked dynamite in a bathing suit.

That's about all there was to this character, an outer beauty that was more than enough to create a lasting global sensation.

Suddenly, men all over the world were ranking the women they knew on a scale of one to ten. Did she measure up to the physical beauty, the "10" that Bo Derek was? Did she qualify as this new sex symbol? Women were no longer seen by realistic standards, and for many men, the majority of women fell far short of their new standards and expectations.

Even sadder, as women, we began to judge ourselves by the same ridiculous standards. Collectively, we started to care more about what we looked like than about who we were. Even worse, we labeled ourselves by this numerical scale, as if a number now defined our worth. To be a "10" meant that we were beautiful on the outside, and that became our perceived point of power. In the process, we lost sight of our inherent beauty and perfection of being, something that exists within all women and is our only real power.

The scale was definitely flawed. It measured only superficial qualities such as our hair, our faces, our bodies, our age, and even the color of our skin.

But it gave no consideration to the beauty that existed within—our real beauty.

As I have grown older and worked with women from all walks of life, I have given much thought to what it means to really be beautiful. I have known women in all shapes and sizes, all ages and races, who have glowed with an inner and outer beauty that is solely and uniquely theirs. This showed me that all women are capable of feeling beautiful and that expressing that beauty is simply a matter of getting in touch with the light within ourselves—our divine light.

That's what the New 10 movement is all about.

The New 10 is a new paradigm for beauty that supports the mind, the body, and the spirit. It encourages all women to be the best we can be, inside and out, by focusing on our hearts, our souls, our spirits, and our bodies … and celebrating them without shame or apology.

In our culture, too many women and teens suffer from eating disorders. And depression is becoming an epidemic among women and teens simply because they don't feel beautiful enough, or beautiful at all, period.

We are collectively obsessed with weight loss, our body types, resisting the natural process of aging, and being good enough according to the unrealistic standards of the old "10" paradigm. We will not even think twice about surgical procedures to improve our looks according to our distorted perceptions of what really is beautiful.

As a child and teen, I was considered plump. I was not popular in school; I was a good student, but not one of the pretty ones. Everybody liked me, I was nice and a great friend to have around, but that was not enough. I was not beautiful—not even close to being a "10."

I also had it beaten into me as a child and teen that I was ugly and fat—even stupid, although my grades proved otherwise. After fifteen years of this horrendous conditioning, I believed it wholeheartedly.

As a young adult I attracted men who reflected back to me my complete lack of self-esteem and my inability to love myself.

This kept me in a twenty-year cycle of abusive and self-degrading marriages, all ending because a part of me knew it shouldn't be this way. Finally, I had had enough. I chose to change my perception of myself and of my life.

My success was the direct result of my taking full responsibility for all that I had created because of my past conditioning and my choosing to no longer be a victim.

I learned to love myself, to find my light within and let it shine. I learned the power of feeling beautiful from the inside out. My path to healing is how and why this book was born. This forty-day program takes you through the processes of my learning, growing, and healing. It is a process of empowerment, surrender, and awakening to your beauty within.

I have grown to see my value as a woman, a value that cannot be judged or diminished by anyone, unless I allow it to be. I have reclaimed my real value as a beautiful woman, from the inside out. This book is also part of my bold expression of that inner beauty.

It is within us all; we simply need to recognize it and let it shine and radiate as far and as wide as we are willing to allow. Please know there are no limits to this except those we place on ourselves.

This book is designed to help you unleash the New 10 inside of you—to celebrate your real beauty and live a more beautiful, authentic life. Over the next forty days, we will learn together how to give of ourselves and to ourselves more freely, accept who we are more easily, and love ourselves more fully and unconditionally.

In the process, our true beauty will come shining through, because as you will learn—just by being our vibrant and authentic selves—we are inherently, perfectly beautiful.

The first section of the book focuses on thinking beautiful thoughts. As within, so without, and it starts with our thoughts. We learn the value of having an open mind, and ways to deal with many fears we all share and emotions that we would normally rather repress than lovingly express.

In this section we will change all of that. You will learn how to transform your mind into one that is powerful, loving, and beautiful.

The second section of the book focuses on our bodies ... on loving, caring for, and accepting them as gifts, as vessels, to house our spirits for the glory of our divine expression of that spirit. Do you love your body? Are you safe in your sexual expression? Do you flaunt your fabulous self? Do you smile?

After this section, your relationship with your body will be renewed and you will find it a joyous experience.

Section three is all about embracing our spirits. Do you trust the universe as friendly and wanting you to be happy? How well do you know yourself as a soul? Do you live according to the truth of your heart? Do you know that you cannot ask for too much but rather that you often ask for too little? Do you enjoy life and laugh when the going gets tough?

At the end of this section you will be free from the restrictions of the ego-personality. This aspect of ourselves serves a wonderful purpose, but we are much more than that, and you will learn to love and embrace and express that part of you with ease and grace.

The last section is all about living an extraordinary life. You will learn to say YES to yourself and to life in a bigger, more transparent way. You will learn the art of patience and staying calm under pressure. You will embrace living a charmed life, free of guilt and apology. You will learn the art of real beauty—the art of you!

On the next page you will find my New 10 Beauty Quotient Quiz. This isn't like most quizzes you've taken before; there are no real "right" or "wrong" answers. It just paints a picture of where you are on your New 10 journey right now.

I invite you to take this quiz before we begin, just to get a sense of where you are. You will have a chance to take it again after our forty days are completed. In the meantime, if you would like a private assessment or to talk further about anything in the book, you can visit my Web site at www.boldlybeautiful.com to schedule an appointment. I would love to hear from you and to personally guide you through this program.

Now, let's get started.

It's going to be an amazing few weeks, beautiful!

THE NEW 10 BEAUTY QUOTIENT QUIZ

You should take this quiz before and after reading the book. There is another copy at the back.

PART ONE: I THINK WITH MY BEAUTIFUL MIND

1. When faced with fear, do you avoid the situation or do you allow yourself to feel it and move through it?
2. When faced with a situation where your integrity and values are in question, do you speak your truth or do you stay silent, thinking that it is easier to do so?
3. On a scale of one to ten, how open minded are you in most situations?
4. When you make a mistake or unintentionally hurt another, do you forgive yourself easily, or do you harbor feelings of guilt?
5. When faced with negative emotions, are you able to express them lovingly, or do you lose control or even keep them hidden inside?
6. When faced with problems, do you allow worry to take over, or do you approach them with a healthy concern?
7. How well on a scale of one to ten do you honor your feelings, even if it means possible rejection from someone else?

8. On a scale of one to ten, how confident are you in who you are and your unique contribution to humanity?

9. Do you live in your comfort zone, or do you allow expansion of your comfort zones on a regular basis as part of your overall evolution and growth?

10. Do you practice harmlessness at all times, or do you find it necessary to get even or get back at someone, even if only occasionally?

PART TWO: I LOVE MY BEAUTIFUL BODY

1. Do you honor the guidance of your body at all times, or do you ignore its promptings to exercise, to eat certain foods or not, and to get rest when needed?

2. Do you take the time daily to affirm that your health is perfect, regardless of appearances? Do you place your focus on health?

3. Are you energetically alive? Do your soul and spirit have the chance to shine through your body and express themselves?

4. Do you breathe deeply, in a focused way, with the intention of increasing your vital life force three times a day?

5. Do you dance like no one is watching?

6. Do you work at maintaining your physical strength through exercise and other activities?

7. Do you feel safe in your sexuality?

8. Do you look in the mirror and *feel beautiful?*

9. Do you flaunt the fabulous aspects of yourself at all times?

10. Do you smile when you are alone?

PART THREE: I EXPRESS MY SPIRIT BOLDLY

1. Do you believe in a benevolent universe, one that is friendly and always working with you for your highest good?
2. Are you connected with your soul? Do you know her unique qualities, favorite colors, fragrances, and desires?
3. Do you believe in your innate ability to be powerful beyond measure at all times, by your simply choosing to be so?
4. Do you lead by example, living by your truth and integrity at all times?
5. Are you grateful for the gifts and blessings bestowed upon you in the present moment each day?
6. Are you comfortable with following your divine and intuitive guidance on a daily basis?
7. Do you respect that your imagination is in part your soul trying to guide you to your highest expression in this lifetime?
8. Do you embrace expansion in all areas of your life, knowing that we are constantly evolving and capable of achieving more than we think we can?
9. Do you romance yourself, light candles for yourself, play love music for yourself, date yourself?
10. Are you able to laugh at life's challenges, knowing that in doing so you are freeing your spirit to provide you with solutions to what are actually lessons we are very capable of learning?

PART FOUR: I LIVE A BOLDLY BEAUTIFUL LIFE

1. Do you strive to become more conscious and aware of your patterns and paradigms?

2. Do you value just being, spending time with yourself and doing nothing?

3. Do you live in the present moment, or are your thoughts always focused on the past or future?

4. Do you take the time to think before you speak, especially in times of deeply felt emotions?

5. Are you willing to allow yourself to age beautifully? Are you aware that it is possible to do so?

6. Are you willing to ask for what you want from others, from yourself, and from the universe?

7. Can you dance with your darkness, knowing that she needs your love and acceptance to express and be the light?

8. Do you have a prosperity consciousness, knowing that God is your source of unlimited wealth and supply in all areas of your life, regardless of appearances to the contrary?

9. Are you able to detach from outcomes and therefore create the space for the universe to manifest with you in an easy and graceful manner?

10. Are you patient? Can you let go and trust and have faith in the divine timing of all things that are meant to be for your highest good?

Our deepest fear is not that we are inadequate. Our deepest fear is that we are powerful beyond measure. It is our light, not our darkness that most frightens us. We ask ourselves, Who am I to be brilliant, gorgeous, talented, fabulous? Actually, who are you not to be? You are a child of God. Your playing small does not serve the world. There is nothing enlightened about shrinking so that other people won't feel insecure around you. We are all meant to shine, as children do. We were born to make manifest the glory of God that is within us. It is not just in some of us; it is in everyone. And as we let our own light shine, we unconsciously give other people permission to do the same. As we are liberated from our own fear, our presence automatically liberates others.

— Marianne Williamson, *A Return to Love*

My Thoughts Are Ugly.
My Thoughts Are Beautiful.

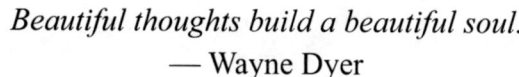

Beautiful thoughts build a beautiful soul.
— Wayne Dyer

You have probably heard the expression "Beauty is only skin deep." Well, I happen to disagree with that statement. Today more than ever, I believe that true beauty starts far deeper than your skin.

I believe beauty starts in the mind.

We all want to feel beautiful. To look in the mirror and like what we see. To face the day feeling confident and comfortable in our own skin. To know we are the best we can be when we walk out the door.

Unfortunately, we may not always feel that way. We may look in the mirror and see only our flaws, completely missing our true beauty, especially if we hold ourselves to unrealistic standards that fail to account for the things that make each one of us unique, special, and beautiful.

But there is something we can do about it right now. We can harness the power of our minds. That is where I'm going to begin our journey.

For the next ten days, we will focus our energy on thinking with our beautiful minds. Since true beauty comes from within, there is no better place to start this transformation. When our minds reflect the beauty of our souls, when we focus on what we love about ourselves and others, our beauty can only grow. We glow with new strength and new confidence. We radiate love and strength. In other words, we are beautiful.

By harnessing the power of your mind—the inside—you transform everything, including the outside. That is why working on the mind is the first step in becoming a New 10.

Are you ready? Then let's go.

Day 1:
I HIDE FROM MY FEARS.
I FACE MY FEARS.

[T]he only thing we have to fear is fear itself.
— Franklin Roosevelt

Welcome to your very first day of our journey together. Together, we are about to embark on an incredible experience that will bring you closer to your true beauty and your true self than you ever thought possible. We are going to begin at the beginning. Today, we're going to talk about fear.

What does fear have to do with beauty? If you're asking that question, you're not alone. When we think about beauty, we usually think about physical things—about being the "right" weight, or having "good hair" or "a pretty face" or "a nice smile."

But there is much more to beauty than how we look on the outside. Being truly beautiful—being the New 10—means embracing who you really, truly are. It means facing yourself without flinching and loving what you see both inside and out. And that takes courage.

Fear is a natural emotion, but it's not a particularly positive one. In most cases, its main purpose seems to be to tell us that we *can't* or *shouldn't* do something. Fear holds us back, it makes us question ourselves, it stops us from being who we truly are, from going after what we really want, from pursuing our ultimate truth.

So when Franklin Roosevelt spoke those immortal words "the only thing we have to fear is fear itself" more than sixty years ago, he wasn't just talking about politics, or war, or the economy.

He was talking about the destructive nature of fear.

That's why, before we can truly begin to access our true beauty, we need to think long and hard about the fears that are holding *us* back.

This is not to say there's something wrong with having fear or feeling afraid—fear is completely and totally normal. What I want you to focus on today, as we embark on this journey together, is how you *handle* that fear. How does your mind work when you are faced with something that makes you feel uncomfortable or uneasy? How do you react the first time you are faced with something new and don't quite know what to make of it?

When you are faced with a fear for the first time, are you able to at least acknowledge to yourself that you are afraid? Many of us cannot. But the first step toward facing our fears is being honest with ourselves and acknowledging that yes, the fear is there. It exists. But it can be dealt with.

Now ask yourself, just because you feel this fear, do you feel any less passionate about what you hope to accomplish? Or is that fear going to stand in your way?

As women, we need to understand and embrace the fact that we are powerful enough to overcome our fears. We have the inner strength necessary to push through to the other side to accomplish our dreams and our goals. By facing and dealing with fear head-on, we clear the way for the work ahead.

I went through this myself in 2006, when I had my first radio show. I was absolutely terrified to hear my own voice on the air, let alone speak my opinions in public. I was raised to believe that "nice girls" kept quiet and didn't share their ideas with the world. What if I was doing the wrong thing? What if no one liked what I said?

But deep down inside, I knew I had the vision to share my truth with a larger audience. I felt that I was being guided to do it. I didn't let fear stand in my way. It wasn't easy, but I pushed through that fear—and actually got invited to be on television! Which of course brought up a whole new set of fears …

What I realized through my radio experience is that as we grow in life, we face more challenges that might seem scary. But the moment we push through that fear is the moment when we really accomplish something. We grow. We change. We become better and stronger.

We become fearless.

So whatever you fear, whatever is holding you back, today is the day to start working to overcome it. It doesn't need to be a superhuman effort; just take it one day at a time. Start with your smallest fear first—something you are confident you can get past—and build from there. It should be an enjoyable process. Once you tackle that small fear, you'll feel energized and empowered to take on a larger one, and a larger one, and a larger one. As you do, you will see that your fears served no purpose other than to hold you back. Eventually, you too will become fearless. And you will be ready to face the unique challenges of the journey ahead.

WHAT REALLY WORKS FOR ME

Since we're starting this journey together today, I want to get one thing clear right off the bat. I am not preaching at you from some perch on high. Every single issue we'll deal with in this book is one that I have experienced, in one form or another, throughout my life. And some of them I still struggle with today.

Fear is one of those issues. Just because I've conquered one fear doesn't mean another one won't pop up along the way! But one of my teachers, Sonia Choquette, has given me an exercise that has really helped me face up to my fears and get past them. It has not only helped me tackle some particularly nasty fears, but also paved the way for me to achieve some of my dreams.

This exercise is called Digging for Gold. Basically, what you do is sit down at your computer, or with a pad of lined paper, and ask yourself this: "If I weren't afraid, I would …" The goal is to write down every single thing that comes to mind. Everything you'd do if fear weren't stopping you, from bungee jumping off a bridge to asking the cute guy in the next cubicle on a date to dying your hair red.

When you have at least 100 ideas (yes, that's a lot, but they don't ALL have to be serious!), read over your list. Then pick three ideas—ideally the things you want to do the most—and do them, one by one.

It might help to start with an idea that scares you less than some of the others. When you tackle that fear, it will give you more confidence in your ability to move through your fear and see that you will be okay and stronger for it. I've also found it really helpful to do this exercise with a friend, so we can share the experience, support each other, and not allow each other to give up. But it's also perfectly fine to do it alone and offer that support to yourself.

Good luck, THINK BIG, and most important, have fun with this!

Day 2:
WHO CARES WHAT I THINK?
I CARE WHAT I THINK.

Don't make me walk when I want to fly.
— Galina Doyla

Welcome to Day 2 of our journey together. Yesterday, we talked about facing our fears, and how pushing through them and overcoming them can help in our quest to achieve true inner and outer beauty. Today, we're going to look a bit more closely at what ranks as a chart-topping fear for a lot of women: speaking your truth.

I want to begin by asking you a very important question. When you are faced with a situation where your values and integrity are in question, what do you do? Are you able to speak your truth comfortably and confidently? Or do you stay silent, thinking that it's probably best to not say anything at all and wait for whatever the incident or issue is to "blow over"?

For many of us, the latter answer is, sadly, more likely to be true. There's no reason to feel bad or beat yourself up about it. To be honest, I am one of many women who grew up believing that opening my mouth and standing up for what I believed in was wrong, unfeminine, and, in fact, ugly. It is not uncommon for women to believe that.

The good news is, I am happy and honored to be able to tell you that it is also completely and totally wrong.

Part of being a fully empowered woman is being able to find the confidence to speak your truth. Please understand, this doesn't mean you have to yell and scream and stamp your feet, put people down, or offend or insult anyone. You can express what you know and feel is right in your heart with conviction and love instead of anger and bullying. That means you do not have to demand that others agree with you, or to insist that you are "right" and they are "wrong."

Being "right" and "winning" is not what speaking your truth is all about.

Speaking your truth means not being afraid—yes, overcoming fear again—to express what is inside of you. It means knowing that what is inside of you is good and true and honest, and that you have a right to express it and a right to be heard. It's knowing at the deepest level that you have *value*.

Finding the voice to speak your truth can be scary or uncomfortable, especially if you're not usually an outspoken person. You might wonder how others will react, or what they will think of you. And to be perfectly honest, you cannot control what others think or feel about you.

All you can do is *be* you.

You can remind yourself to face situations with both strength *and* gentleness. You can remind yourself that when your values or integrity are on the line, staying true to who you are and what you believe actually allows your beauty to shine through. Nothing is more beautiful than a woman with the confidence and grace to live her truth and convictions.

So start small. Promise yourself that, beginning just once a day, you will stand up for yourself in one situation. You will say no when you want to, instead of saying yes. You will take one moment to place your values before someone else's desires or opinions. You will be true to yourself, no matter what. And you will discover the secret of speaking your truth. Once you start, it only gets easier.

As you stand up for yourself more and more, you will become more comfortable expressing your opinions. Your friends, loved ones, and coworkers will become more accustomed to hearing them from you. And you will become more empowered.

Learning to speak for yourself can help you find the inner strength to build stronger boundaries where you might once have let people walk all over you or take advantage of you. Part of speaking your truth is realizing you have a right to things. You have a right to live in a way that feels true and natural and blessed for you.

As with anything, the more you practice, the easier speaking your truth will get. Your self-confidence will grow as you make and honor this important commitment to yourself. You'll find yourself growing stronger and more confident every day as you find you're more in control of situations.

By really honoring and valuing your integrity and your value system, you can unlock the beauty that's deep within you. That will go a long way toward helping you become the New 10 that you aim to be.

That journey continues tomorrow. …

WHAT REALLY WORKS FOR ME

It's natural to worry about what other people think of us. We want to be liked. We want to be loved. And we certainly don't want other people going around talking behind our backs. I know I don't!

But worrying about what other people think can stifle us from expressing our own truth. I knew this was something I needed to overcome, so a few years ago, I was taught a sentence to use if ever I got caught up in the thoughts and opinions of others to the point where

I was invalidating my own truth. It says, very simply, "It is none of my business what other people think of me."

When you think about it, it really is true. Other people's thoughts are their business, not ours. Not only do we have no control over them but we have no RIGHT to them, really. Just like no other person has a right to know my thoughts (unless I tell them, like I'm telling you right now), or your thoughts.

I use this as my mantra. Whenever I am worried about speaking my truth, I repeat it to remind myself that whatever people think of me is their business. It's what I think of myself that truly matters.

I hope you'll try it. It really does work!

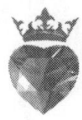

Day 3:
MY MIND IS CLOSED.
MY MIND IS OPEN.

Twenty years from now you will be more disappointed by the things you didn't do than by the ones you did do. So throw off the bowlines. Sail away from the safe harbor. Catch the trade winds in your sail. Explore. Dream. Discover.
— Mark Twain

Welcome to Day 3 of our journey together. Today will help you get your heart and soul ready for all the new experiences that you are going to have over the next thirty-seven days as you work toward becoming a New 10.

Because today is all about opening your mind.

If I asked you if you consider yourself an open-minded person, chances are your answer would be yes. After all, you're reading this book. You've already opened your mind to the idea of looking at and experiencing beauty in a new way. You're at least toying with the idea of doing the work outlined in these chapters—work designed to take you to a place far different from where you are right now. So there has to be at least some open-mindedness there.

Which is a very good thing, because when it comes to unlocking your full beauty potential, open-mindedness is far more important than you might think.

Before we go on, I want you to really, seriously think about this subject. Ask yourself, on a scale of one to ten, one being the lowest, ten being the highest, how open you are to new ideas, to new situations, to change, to growth. When faced with something new, do you jump in with both feet or do you hang back, unwilling or unable to move forward?

If you tend more toward the second category, now is the time to try to let go, just a little, and open yourself up to new ways of seeing and doing things.

The reason is simple. When we close ourselves off from new thoughts, new ideas, and new experiences, we limit ourselves. We fail to grow. And our true beauty is almost smothered under a protective blanket that stands between us and the world around us.

Becoming a New 10 means shedding that blanket and being open to everything the world has to offer.

It means experiencing everything that we can, from sampling new foods and trying new activities to approaching new people and doing things in new ways. Every time we open ourselves to a new experience, it enriches us, adding more depth to our beings and more layers to our souls. In other words, it makes us more beautiful.

If, when you think long and hard and honestly about how open-minded you are, you find you're only at a five or less on our scale of one to ten, don't despair. But do try to do something about it. Try to boost your open-mindedness quotient to seven, or even eight.

As with all things, you might want to start slowly. Try a new food. Take a class or read a book in a subject you haven't found the time or energy to look into. Talk to a stranger. Instead of automatically saying "no," or "I can't," say "yes" and "I can"—even if it's just to little things. Remember, every new experience helps you grow. And each time you grow, you grow more beautiful.

Please understand that this does NOT mean saying yes to something that you know is wrong, or dangerous, or unhealthy, simply because it is "new." We can all trust our common sense to tell us when our resistance to something comes not from closed-mindedness, but from healthy self-preservation. There are some things in life that it is perfectly fine to say no to!

However, we can also say no to limiting thoughts and beliefs. We can let go of preconceived ideas. We can free ourselves to really think outside the box and be willing to change our perspective on ourselves, the people we know, and the world around us.

Personally, trying to think on a higher level helps me open my mind. I try to see myself and everyone around me in a more universal way, on a more global level, as part of the same beautiful world. I want my thoughts and actions to help me make a difference in the world, to make it a better place, and by opening my mind, I know that I can do it. about five years ago You can do it too.

As you continue your journey to becoming a New 10, don't be afraid to open your beautiful mind to all the amazing possibilities in the world around you. You never know what you might find or where the road might take you when you start to say yes.

We'll continue down that road tomorrow.

WHAT REALLY WORKS FOR ME

If you're like most people, chances are you've made a New Year's resolution before. And chances are probably almost as good that you've broken it. Well, I've found a way around that. Instead of making New Year's resolutions, I make very specific and clear New Year's intentions.

I make a firm and unflinching commitment to doing everything that the universe guides me to do, be, and become, fearlessly.

Every day, I remind myself of that commitment. And every day, I become more and more passionate about seeking out and spotting new and different experiences, allowing new doors to open, widening my vistas and embracing change. It's all simply a matter of making that commitment to seek out what I might have turned away from or ignored in the past.

Honestly, my life has not been the same since—it's been a continual series of new adventures, and I have grown a lot throughout the process. Again, I am NOT PERFECT. I have had to make an effort at this, but it has paid off a thousand fold. I know in my heart that you can do it too. Make that commitment to be open to the new and the different … and don't wait until New Year's. Start today!

Day 4:
FAILURE WILL DESTROY ME.
FAILURE MAKES ME STRONGER.

*Our greatest glory is not in never failing, but
in rising up every time we fall.*
— Ralph Waldo Emerson

Welcome to the fourth day of our forty-day quest to redefine beauty. If you've been following along with me so far, ideally you've made an effort to face a fear or two, speak your truth, and open your mind to a new idea or experience.

Maybe you're already starting to feel a change inside of you as you subtly shift the way you do things. Maybe you've experienced new sides of yourself and felt a connection to your soul you hadn't felt before.

Then again, maybe things haven't gone exactly the way you'd hoped.

Maybe, when that moment came to speak your truth, you stayed silent instead.

Maybe, when you were presented with an opportunity to try something new, you went with the tried-and-true, comfortable choice instead.

Or maybe you were working on overcoming your fear of spiders, and you saw a spider in the bathroom and completely freaked out. If it was a big one, I can relate!

It doesn't matter. It's absolutely, completely, and perfectly okay. Because I want you to repeat something, something that is very, very important, right now.

There are no mistakes.

Say it again. There. Are. No. Mistakes.

Look at it this way. We are all—each one of us—souls learning lessons at this school, sort of an earth school called life. Along the way, as we go through the process of learning our lessons, it's completely normal and natural to make mistakes, unintentionally and unconsciously. In fact, we wouldn't be learning if we didn't.

Remember when you were a little girl, and you first learned the alphabet? You didn't automatically know all twenty-six letters in a row. You probably got it wrong quite a few times. Maybe you couldn't get past *R* or you mixed up *K* and *J*. But those mistakes were part of the process as you slowly, systematically learned your letters.

The same is true of almost anything and everything you have ever learned, from how to tie your shoes to how to use the computer. The bottom line is that making mistakes is essential to learning. And if mistakes are an essential part of learning, then we really shouldn't regard them as mistakes at all. They are simply a necessary part of the learning process.

Accept right now that you will not master everything you try immediately. You will not be perfect. And in the process of making these completely normal and natural mistakes, you may possibly hurt another person, or even hurt yourself. Remind yourself that this is okay. It's part of learning. It's part of growing. It's part of life.

In fact, the one lesson that you absolutely MUST learn—although chances are you will not be perfect in this area either—is to forgive yourself. I'll say that again too. Forgive yourself.

The next time you make a mistake, and you will, don't beat yourself up about it. Instead, try this little exercise. Take a deep breath. Step back from the moment. And say to yourself, "You know what? That was a lesson and I'm going to learn that lesson, and I'm going to forgive myself in the process because that's what I'm here for."

It really is that simple. By releasing yourself from the pressure to be perfect—by reminding yourself that every time you make a mistake, it means you are learning that much more—you free yourself to learn what you need to learn, try what you need to try, and even, shocking as it might sound, to fail where you need to fail.

There is no failure, really. There are no mistakes, really. There are just steps on the journey as you grow closer and closer to becoming that New 10.

Remember, change is never easy. So today, I really want to congratulate you for coming this far, for taking this chance, and for giving yourself this gift. I want to encourage you to let go and learn your lessons gracefully. If you can learn to forgive yourself as easily and as quickly as you can, you will free yourself more than you can possibly imagine.

Imagine what you can accomplish without that little voice inside of you putting you down and telling you that you "can't."

Imagine how far you can go if you don't get in your own way.

That's what learning to forgive yourself is all about. By giving yourself permission to make mistakes and fail, you're really giving yourself permission to grow.

That's how you become a New 10.

WHAT REALLY WORKS FOR ME

When I make a mistake, I don't punish myself for failing. Ever. In fact, I celebrate my mistake, because it means I have learned something important. I reward myself for the experience, for having the courage to try and to fail, and of course, for getting back up again when I fall (this is the important part—you can't just lie there on the ground!).

The first time I did this, I made a conscious decision to count how many times I had fallen and how many times I had gotten back up. I saw a pattern. I saw how never giving up made me a stronger, better, wiser person. About five years ago I celebrated myself and my successes. (This was a HUGE celebration, as I have gotten back up many, many times!)

I decided that I wanted to live a life of excellence, and to do that, I know I must try things and I must fail in order to learn and to grow. It's part of the process. I slowly gave up perfectionist tendencies and attitudes and replaced them with states of grace and acceptance for whatever happens along the way.

I fully encourage you to do the same thing. Take an inventory of all the times you've fallen, and instead of beating yourself up, treat yourself to a celebration. Look back at all the times you've picked yourself up from failure and disappointment, and celebrate how much you've learned from those experiences. Most of all, give yourself permission to keep trying and, yes, even to keep failing—because every time you do, you grow that much more.

Day 5:
ANGER IS BAD.
ANGER IS HEALTHY.

The oyster turns into pearl the sand which annoys it.
— Sidney Newton Bremer

It's now Day 5 on our journey toward becoming a New 10, and time to look more closely at something you might not feel very comfortable talking about, or even thinking about. No, I'm not talking about sexuality (although we will get to that later!). I'm talking about something a lot of women find even harder to deal with: negative emotions.

Let's be honest. We all experience negative emotions sometimes. Maybe we get angry at our children when they don't listen. Maybe we feel rejected when our husbands or partners forget a special day or choose to spend time with their friends instead of with us. Maybe we even feel jealous of our girlfriends when they lose weight or get a promotion or start a new romance.

Even if you've never personally experienced any of these examples, you have no doubt experienced pain, envy, anger, sadness, and a wide range of other negative emotions throughout your life. You wouldn't be human if you didn't.

The issue here is not whether or not you experience negative emotions.

The issue is how you deal with them.

Think about it for a minute. When faced with a negative emotion, what do you do? Do you say nothing, try to feel nothing, and squash those negative feelings down inside of you, willing them to just go away?

Are you more likely to lash out in the heat of the moment, possibly hurting those around you or saying things you wind up regretting later?

Or do you allow yourself to fully feel and experience your emotion, calm yourself down, and then actually talk about your feelings?

It's probably fairly obvious that the third choice is the "right" answer. However, reacting calmly and rationally to negative emotions isn't always our first instinct.

This is completely normal—as women, we are all emotional beings. It's so, so important for us to accept that fact. Emotions are simply a natural part of who we are. And it's natural that, since we don't live in a perfect world, we will face experiences that hurt, sadden, anger, and disappoint us.

We are going to be faced with negative emotions.

Many of us have been raised to feel that negativity of any kind is a bad thing, so when we feel a negative emotion coming on, we use all of our energy to try to stop ourselves from feeling it. To the outside world, we may "look" fine, and this may be what we want. But squashing your emotions is not good for you on the *inside*. Those negative feelings will manifest themselves in some way—in health problems, in depression, even in your appearance. Keeping them locked away inside of you actually gives them more power. So although you may be more comfortable hiding negative feelings, this ultimately isn't the best choice.

It may be physically healthier to let those emotions go, but simply blowing up at people is not the best way to deal with them. At the very least, losing your cool can be embarrassing. At the worst, you can hurt people, or even hurt yourself. You can end up using that negativity as a weapon, which then brings negativity into someone else's life—and you know you don't want to do that.

This is why it is so important for us to learn to harness our emotions. To take a deep breath and really try to center ourselves when we sense a bad feeling coming on. Once we take a moment to process what we're feeling, we can express it in a calm, rational way, without hurting other people or ourselves in the process.

This is not the same as stifling our emotions and pretending they are not there. By dealing honestly with our emotions, we build our emotional strength on a really spiritual level. It helps us live in integrity with who we are.

I really encourage you to not stuff your negative emotions, but to face them and deal with them honestly. They're real, and they're valid.

Another thing you can do to process and deal with negative emotions is write about them in a journal. This is especially helpful for women who don't feel comfortable expressing their emotions in public. By writing about what you feel, you can express yourself however you want to—and nobody else ever has to see it. Meanwhile, the act of thinking and writing about your feelings will release them from your body and your mind. This keeps those negative feeling from getting "stuck" and gaining control over your life. It releases them back into the universe. It lets them go.

Remember, on their own, negative emotions aren't bad. They are just what they are. What matters is how you deal with them. And there is a way to work through them.

Will you deal with them perfectly every time? Probably not. But remember, there are no mistakes. And as you practice and learn to handle your emotions, you will find yourself feeling stronger, more in control, and more in touch with who you are. Which is a very beautiful thing.

WHAT REALLY WORKS FOR ME

It may sound a little cliché, but honestly, I scream into pillows when I feel really angry or frustrated. It's great because no one can hear me, and I can scream as loud and as long as I want or need to. It might sound silly, but the act of screaming—of acknowledging just how angry and frustrated I am and letting it out—releases all that negative energy from my physical body. Once it's gone, I am ready to move through the day and respond normally to people and situations instead of reacting to them through that prism of anger and suppressed emotions. That is also referred to as a "bad mood." My motto is, why hold on to it when you can get rid of it?

I've also learned to see the emotions in other people being reflected back to me. This might sound complicated, but it isn't. If people react to me warily, like they're afraid to get too close, I take this as a sign that I am putting out some negative emotions I might not even be aware of. I take a moment to accept and acknowledge those feelings privately—and yes, if I have to, I make time to scream into a pillow! The important thing is to release these feelings through allowing them and accepting them.

Believe me, I know it can be really uncomfortable dealing with our negative feelings. But I have learned that it is necessary, and it is for you too. You will get to know the feelings of joy, love, and peace as your reward.

Day 6:
I ALWAYS WORRY.
I NEVER WORRY.

God, grant me the serenity to accept the things that I cannot change; The courage to change the things I can; And the wisdom to know the difference.
— Dr. Reinhold Niebuhr

If you're like a lot of women, you might have read today's chapter heading and immediately thought, "Why not?"

Which is why our sixth day is going to be devoted to talking about worry.

As women, we are expert worriers. Many of us tend to worry quite a lot. We worry about our loved ones, about our jobs, about our appearance. We worry what other people think of us. We worry about random things like swine flu and plane crashes and recession and war.

In fact, some of us are such devoted, dedicated, professional worriers that when we're not worrying about one thing, we immediately attach that worry to something else.

It takes time. It takes energy. It takes commitment.

But most of us never ask ourselves this very important question: What does all this worrying accomplish?

The answer, if you're like most of us, is probably nothing.

In fact, if you allow worry to consume you when you've got issues and problems, what tends to happen is that you spend all your time *worrying* about those issues and problems but very little time actually *solving* them. Because worry isn't constructive. It isn't about finding solutions. It's about thinking, over and over, about *the worst possible thing that can happen.* And then imagining it happening over and over again.

The worst part is that while you're thinking about that horrible, horrible thing that might happen, something that really is kind of horrible is happening. When we worry, we actually stop ourselves from finding solutions. All that "what if this happens" and "what if that happens" in our minds gets in the way and blocks the universe from trying to help us resolve the real issue.

More often than not, the answers we are looking for are right there in front of us. But when we get so caught up in the worry and the emotions surrounding that worry, we literally can't hear what the universe is trying to tell us. And when that divine guidance that's so readily available comes to us, we won't even recognize it, even if it hits us right over the head. All that worrying will simply drown it out.

It's not that we don't know worrying is bad—we do. We've all heard that it causes everything from wrinkles to gray hair to ulcers. It's just that it's so hard to let worry go. Many of us worry that if we don't worry (which basically says it all right there, doesn't it?), we somehow aren't being responsible. We won't do what we need to do, we'll let something slip, we'll mess up somehow.

I want to assure you that absence of worry does not mean absence of responsibility of any kind. You are absolutely allowed to have a healthy concern for issues like your finances, your children's health, or anything else that's important in your life. It's not just normal and natural, it's necessary.

The difference is all in the language. If you say that you "have a concern" instead of saying you're "worried," you're letting the universe know that you're not just dwelling on the problem, but are open to solutions. You're putting out the fact that something is on your mind and asking for help.

And then—and this is the hard part—you let it go. You put your concern out there, and you let it go. You do what you need to do, and you trust the universe to do the rest.

If you are a person who tends to worry, it's probably not practical to decide you're just "not going to worry" anymore. But by exchanging that worry for a healthy concern, you put yourself back in control of the situation. Instead of simply waiting for disaster to befall you, you will make sure that your mind is open to guidance and open to the wisdom that will help you through. That wisdom is always there. You just need to quiet the voices in your head to hear it sometimes.

The best part is, when you allow yourself access to that wisdom, when you give yourself the space you need to find the solutions you want, you feel empowered. Do you know what happens then? You wind up feeling good about yourself. And that's what this is really all about. Finding strength you didn't know you had. Listening to wisdom you didn't know was there.

And always, always growing.

WHAT REALLY WORKS FOR ME

Okay, you've got me on a tough one here. To be completely honest, this is an area where I am still learning every day and growing into a more faithful existence. I have a lot of hopes and dreams, and I'm sure you do too, and it can be difficult to live in the now instead of constantly wondering and worrying about what might happen.

I can tell you from experience that meditation really, really helps me when I need to hold my own counsel. It helps take the focus off whatever thoughts are rattling around in my head and helps me find my center and reconnect with God and the universe. It reminds me that this day, this moment, is just one of many, and that the universe is looking out for me, and that I will be okay. I know in the bottom of my heart that this will work for you too. Meditation is a real gift.

There are still times when I need guidance from another person—when I really want and need another opinion from someone who can view my problem or question objectively. During times like these, I turn to my trusted friends at www.12Listen.com and www.12Angel.com. They are all excellent advisers and healers, and their advice really comes in handy when I'm facing an important decision or issue.

Remember, you can't banish worry by magic, and you shouldn't expect yourself to. Instead of expecting yourself to go from a place of worry to a place of total freedom from worry in one fell swoop, try going for a "healthy concern" to find the peace of mind that you richly deserve.

Day 7:
IF I'M REJECTED, I'LL DIE!
IF I'M REJECTED, I WILL SURVIVE.

*Let me pray not to be sheltered from dangers,
but to be fearless in facing them. Let me not beg for
the stilling of my pain, but for the heart to conquer it.*
— Tagore

Rejection. The word alone can strike fear in the hearts of women—not to mention men—around the world. In fact, so many people live their lives in abject fear of rejection that they avoid saying or doing anything that might result in their being rejected, which severely limits what they can do with their lives, since rejection is a fact of life.

Fear of rejection is a big problem—so big that, even though I've already dedicated a day to facing your fears, I'd like to spend the eighth day of our journey together exploring rejection a little more deeply.

Nobody likes being rejected. It can be embarrassing, it's usually disappointing, and sometimes it even hurts. All in all, it's just not a lot of fun. But although rejection is almost by definition unpleasant, some of us deal with it much better than others do.

Believe it or not, there are people out there who accept rejection as such a natural part of life that it barely registers with them. They just keep going.

Then there are others who view any rejection as a condemnation of their deepest self. When they are rejected, they find it so devastating that they live in fear of it happening again.

Most of us fall somewhere in between the two extremes. It's important to understand where you fit on the scale—and to really get a handle on how rejection affects you.

Think for a moment about how you handle rejection. Do you honor your feelings when things don't go your way, or do you beat yourself up and blame yourself?

And more important, do you let the fear of rejection stand in your way? Does the fear of what other people might say or do or think prevent you from moving forward with your goals and plans and dreams?

Being able to handle rejection is so, so important to becoming a New 10. If you take risks in life, if you put yourself out there and go for what you really want, chances are very high that at some point along the way, you will be rejected. Someone, at some point, is going to say no to you. If you let that crush your spirit, if you let it destroy you, then you let it destroy your chance to grow.

We need to learn how to not let that happen.

But how do we do that?

We can demystify rejection and take away the power it seems to hold over us. As women, we want to please everyone all the time. We want everyone to like us, to want us, to approve of us. So when someone turns us down for something that matters to us, we tend to take that rejection personally.

But more often than not, rejection has nothing to do with you and everything to do with the other person involved. The timing might not be right. The chemistry might not be right. Or it just might not be what the universe wants. If we trust in the universe, trust in ourselves, and trust that things really do happen for a reason, then rejection becomes what it should be: a way to weed out people and situations that aren't right for us. In other words, it is just part of the natural process of life.

Remember how, on a journey when you are learning and growing, there are no mistakes? Well, in a life in which you take chances and try new things, there really is no rejection. As the old saying goes, you can't please everybody, so you've got to please yourself. If you live in constant fear of rejection, chances are you're spending far too much time and energy trying to please other people instead of being true to yourself. The only person you really need to please is you. That means no one else can really reject you.

So don't let fear of rejection hold you back. If you are going to become everything that you are meant to be and reach your full potential as a woman and as a human being, there is only one person you truly need to listen to, and that is you. You need to listen to your heart and soul, and you need to honor what they tell you.

Life is not a dress rehearsal. This is it, and you know what? We are all meant to shine. We are meant to be the stars of our own lives. So know that I honor you in all the work you are doing to overcome your fears, especially the fear of rejection. When you refuse to give others power over you and to give your fears power over you, you gain that much more power for yourself.

That's a very important part of this journey.

WHAT REALLY WORKS FOR ME

I have made a promise to myself: I am willing to be rejected in all circumstances if it means that I am staying on my path and following my heart. That means I don't shy away from situations where I might be rejected. I remind myself that, whatever the outcome, I am pursuing this thing because I am following my truth. And if I happen to be rejected, it is not because there is something wrong with me. It is because the universe wants something else for me.

This gave me the strength to let go of a marriage that did not support my true nature. The process of divorce was very trying and I was challenged at every turn, rejected with every offer for truth and freedom. But those rejections were my road map—they directed me where I was supposed to go. I did not give up. I kept trying and kept working, and although I was still rejected, I found my way through.

By being very clear about what I truly value and what I need to feel happy and fulfilled, I can take a stand for what I want and value. Sometimes this leads to rejection. But I believe that my happiness is my own responsibility and no one else's, so a rejection simply means that there would have been no happiness for me in that situation anyway. In that way, I view rejection as a gift that keeps me from wasting my time and my energy on things that ultimately will not work for me.

The only rejection that really matters is the rejection of ourselves. I have learned to always accept myself, and urge you to accept yourself as well. Beyond that, rejection is a gift, something that shows you are truly on your path and being guided toward exactly what is right for you.

Day 8:
I AM WORTHLESS.
I AM PRICELESS.

Life is no brief candle to me. It is a sort of splendid torch which I have got a hold of for the moment, and I want to make it burn as brightly as possible before handing it on to future generations.
— George Bernard Shaw

It's been said that the most attractive part of a woman isn't great hair or a perfect body, but confidence. But for some of us, feeling confident is not all that easy. Many women just don't feel good about themselves, no matter how hard they try. We feel that we don't look right, that we aren't achieving enough, that we aren't "good enough" to be worthy of much of anything.

For Day 8, we're going to tackle this lack of confidence head-on. We all have a reason to be confident deep, deep inside of us. We just need to access it and bring it into the light.

So here it is.

Whoever you are, whatever you do, right at this moment, you are making a contribution to the world. And you need to celebrate that.

If you are a president of a company, or a star athlete, or a professional entertainer, chances are you already know and feel in your heart that you are making a contribution to the world. When your job commands respect, when you are told by society that you are "important," the idea that you're making a contribution usually comes with the territory. If you aren't a particularly confident person and you fit into this category, remind yourself of your success and your contribution to the world. Remember that you earned it and deserve it, and feel good and confident about your accomplishments.

If you are a teacher, nurse, police officer, firefighter, or someone else who helps others for a living, you probably know on some level that the work you do is helping humanity. You probably understand that you are also making an important contribution to the world. This is definitely something to celebrate and feel good about. People like you are so essential to our world and our society that you should know, every day, how truly important and special you are. You need to connect with this part of yourself, especially when you're feeling low—it has great power to remind you to feel confident.

But what if you are a stay-at-home mother? Can you feel confident in that?

My answer to you is simple. What could possibly be more important than teaching and growing the next generation of humanity? Our children are going to inherit our world. Raising them to be strong (and confident!) by showing them that they are loved and cared for is the best possible preparation for the challenges of life. That is a definite contribution, and definitely something to feel good about.

Of course, not all of us are parents. Not all of us are even employed. Some of us work at jobs we're not particularly passionate about. The good news is, your contribution doesn't necessarily have to come from your job. It comes from *who you are*.

Whether you're a good friend, an amazing cook, or even just a person who shares a smile with a stranger, you add something to this world. We all do. We all have individual ways of making a contribution.

The next step is to celebrate that contribution. Once you identify what you're giving to the world, you can develop your inner confidence and a passion for that contribution that will enable you to take it to the next level. As you grow in your contribution, everyone you know, and even people you don't know, will benefit. The universe will benefit from the fact that you're operating at your highest potential and giving something to the world.

Most important, you will be able to shine and grow and contribute at higher and higher levels. As you do, you'll expand your consciousness, expand your ability to contribute, and even expand what you have to give. You will become more confident and feel more beautiful than you ever have. When you're feeling confident and sharing your gifts with the world, whatever they may be, you can't help but exude the natural beauty of who you are inside.

We all are intrinsically beautiful when we live at that deeper level. And this is the level we're aiming to reach—the level where every one of us is a New 10.

So whoever you are and whatever you do, think about what you contribute to the world around you, and concentrate on and celebrate that part of yourself. This is where your true beauty begins.

WHAT TRULY WORKS FOR ME

The best way for me to grow my self-confidence is to always treat myself like I am special. That means I am loving and true to my inner wisdom and guidance. I celebrate my beauty and the perfection of being—imperfections and all! And I do my best to take care of myself, inside and out, because I deserve to be treated well. When I do those things, I feel great and my confidence soars.

Most important, it's about being kind to myself, remembering to have fun, and forgiving myself when I slip up. Because we all slip up!

For me, self-confidence does not come from being perfect. It comes from living honestly, experiencing the joy that comes from life, and loving myself, imperfections and all.

It comes from living a life that I can be proud of and striving to be the person I want to be. Even when I miss the mark, I feel good about myself for trying, for always being willing to take the risk, go the extra mile, live in integrity, and be true to myself.

I promise, if you live in integrity and honor the beautiful person you are, your confidence will soar!

Day 9:
I LIKE TO FEEL SAFE.
I LIKE TO FEEL CHALLENGED.

Far better it is to dare mighty things, to win glorious triumphs, even though checkered by failure, than to rank with those poor spirits who neither enjoy much nor suffer much, because they live in the gray twilight that knows not victory nor defeat.
— Theodore Roosevelt

Hello and welcome to Day 9 of our journey together. I hope you have been enjoying the steps so far as you grow toward your future as a New 10. Ideally you've been able to take a few risks, try a few new things, look at life and yourself in a new way—and maybe you've even started to notice a transformation in yourself.

Of course, growth isn't always easy. It takes work and practice. One thing I've learned on my own journey is that the times when I seem to grow the most as a woman and as a human being usually require me to leave my comfort zone.

We all have a comfort zone—that place where we know that we'll be okay and feel safe no matter what. Those comfort zones tend to vary from person to person. Some people have very limited comfort zones and basically allow themselves only a small range of experiences.

Others are perfectly open to new things in some areas, but are far less comfortable taking chances in other parts of their lives.

For example, maybe you love traveling to new places and trying new things, but you haven't changed your hairstyle or makeup since high school or college. That's an example of staying in a comfort zone. Maybe you keep up with all the latest fashion trends, but you stay in a job that you find boring and soul stifling. Or maybe you've taken a huge risk by starting your own business, but you still vacation in the same place at the same time every year.

None of this is particularly strange, or even wrong. As human beings, we all like to be comfortable. We all have areas of our lives where that need for comfort takes charge. Although we may be interested in the idea of trying new things and having new experiences, we might put them off until another day when we feel braver, more rested, more ready.

Well, it's time to get ready. Because today is all about expanding your comfort zone.

We all step out of our comfort zones from time to time, because whoever we are, we face situations that require us to leave them momentarily. There are occasions when we do it out of necessity, times we feel uncharacteristically bold or free, and other times when we do things we wouldn't normally do simply to go along with someone else's desires.

Expanding your comfort zone is a little different. Instead of taking a giant but momentary leap and doing something that's completely and totally NOT you, expanding your comfort zone is more gentle ... and more lasting. As we grow and become more empowered and more awakened to our true, beautiful selves, our comfort zones simply have to grow along with us.

Today is about pushing the boundaries a little bit, stretching a little bit beyond the place where you would normally stop yourself. It's asking a tiny bit more of yourself in a way that enables you to discover, slowly but surely, that there is more to you than you might imagine. And that you can do more than you ever thought possible.

Sometimes, the areas where we most need to expand our comfort zones are the areas we are also most resistant to. These are areas of our lives that we need to pay special attention to, because often getting past these blocks is exactly what our souls want and need us to do, especially if staying in that comfort zone is actually blocking us from becoming who we need to be.

Take a look at those areas of your life and open yourself to the fact that your soul may be guiding you to pay attention. Try to listen to your soul and let yourself expand beyond your comfort zone, even if it's only a little.

The more you work at it, the more you expand your comfort zone, the more your mind-set is going to expand. Your whole world will open up to new possibilities, new opportunities, and new people. You will find that, just like everything I have introduced so far in this book, expanding your comfort zone gets easier and the more determined you are the more successful you are.

Keep going. Keep moving forward. Keep learning and growing. The more you do, the closer you'll get to your new life as a New 10.

And that's something I know you will be comfortable with.

WHAT REALLY WORKS FOR ME

Here's an unusual concept for you. I have chosen to become very comfortable with being uncomfortable. I have trained my mind to see discomfort as positive. I actively seek out situations that will push me beyond my boundaries. In fact, if I get too comfortable, I start to get restless. This means I'm not learning, not growing, essentially not living. So I am constantly in a state of "going for it"—looking for the new and untried and setting my sights on it. This has, in turn, fostered tremendous growth on my part. And it has taught me to actually enjoy feeling uncomfortable.

By living this way, I have let go of being a victim of life's circumstances and chosen to be a victor in the fulfillment of my wishes and dreams instead. I make my life happen. Does it always work? Of course not. But it's always a new adventure, and I am always, always growing.

So take some baby steps and start expanding your comfort zone. I promise it does get easier!

Day 10:
THE WORLD IS MY ENEMY.
THE WORLD IS MY FRIEND.

It is easy enough to be pleasant, when life flows along like a song, but the man worthwhile is the man with a smile, when everything goes dead wrong.
— Author Unknown

For the past nine days, we've been working together on your beautiful mind, helping it expand, grow, and access your true inner beauty. We've talked about fear and rejection, speaking out and coping with negative feelings, confidence and comfort zones—all of which are terms and concepts you're probably familiar with.

Well, today, I want to close out this section by talking about something that may sound a bit more strange and foreign to you: the idea of harmlessness.

If I asked you if you practice harmlessness in your everyday life, you might not understand what I mean. Does it mean not killing spiders or eating meat? Does it mean letting other people walk all over you? What exactly does it mean to be harmless?

Essentially, harmlessness is based in being aware of your reactions to situations and to others, and, in all cases, striving to do no harm in everything that you say and do.

Harmlessness is not the same as helplessness. You can and should still respond when you need to, you can still stand up for yourself, you can still have boundaries, and you can still be powerful. Practicing harmlessness does not diminish any of this. Harmlessness is about the *way* we approach these situations, and about approaching them in a way that actually gives us even more power.

When we approach others from a place of confidence and strength, we have the power to treat them gently, without anger, without threats, without causing them any needless pain. We don't need to lash out or be nasty or dramatic or emotional, because we are coming from a place of peace and calm, where we know we are doing the right thing.

This not only prevents us from hurting others but even more important, prevents us from hurting ourselves. We cannot hurt another person without ultimately hurting ourselves even more.

When we are able to approach everyone in our lives from a place of love, calm, and grace, negative emotions and experiences don't stop our inner beauty from shining through. In fact, we become even more beautiful as we learn to find that calm, steady center in our souls and to always operate from there, no matter what the situation may be.

Imagine how amazing it would feel to go through life with that level of confidence and self-control—where you are not only strong enough to ask for what you want but able to see the other person's perspective and respect it at all times. It might sound like a lot, but it really is simple. It's all about remembering that no matter what situation you find yourself in, the only reaction you can control is your own. When you control that reaction, when you ask yourself to operate from your soul and be the best person you can be, that grace and beauty shines on everyone around you.

Is this easy to do? Of course not. But the results are so, so worth it. Whatever sort of healing you might need to do to be able to get to that place—whether it's energy healing or energy balancing or just taking a deep breath to calm yourself in difficult situations—I really encourage you to do it. And to work steadily toward a place where you can find the strength to be gentle and kind.

Practicing harmlessness is the final piece of the puzzle of your beautiful mind. It's integral to feeling beautiful and to exuding that intrinsic inner beauty that exists deep inside of you. Master this technique and you will be well on your way to your shining, beautiful future as a New 10.

WHAT REALLY WORKS FOR ME

The best way I know to practice harmlessness is to share as much love with the world as I can, every single day. I love to practice random acts of kindness—doing something nice for a stranger, surprising a friend or relative. I love to give, to tip generously, to give presents, to bring smiles to people's faces. It's so easy—almost effortless, really—to put myself in a positive frame of mind by giving. When I see the joy on other people's faces, I know I am bringing something positive to the world just by being in it.

My challenge has been to be as kind and giving to myself as I am with others. This is an area I have to work on. But I am learning to treat myself to those little smiles and special moments the same way I treat other people. It's hard to feel negative when you're treating yourself to a latte, or filling a vase with your favorite flower. I do this with myself, and it helps me relate to the world around me in the most positive way possible. It goes beyond spending money on myself. It also means being gentle with myself when I fall, picking myself up, and giving myself the support and appreciation I need.

Ask yourself whether you really appreciate yourself for all that you do. Start doing no harm with yourself first. … You do count!

I HATE MY BODY.
I LOVE MY BODY.

> *The best and most beautiful things in the*
> *world cannot be seen, nor touched ...*
> *but are felt in the heart.*
> — Helen Keller

Our bodies do so much for us. They embody our hearts and our souls. They allow us to experience all that life has to offer. They are not only the vessels for our true beauty but are totally and absolutely necessary to our existence on this earth.

However, despite how important our bodies are to us, many of us aren't very nice to our bodies.

For many women, "body image issues" are a fact of life. We wish our bodies looked different—often like unrealistic, airbrushed images of teenage models in magazines. And we beat ourselves up when they don't.

We wish our bodies felt different—free of disease and aches and pains, and forever young and strong.

Some of us even wish our bodies *behaved* differently—that they were free from the appetites and urges that every normal woman has.

That's why I want to dedicate the second part of our journey together to accepting and loving our beautiful bodies and doing all we can for them.

For the next ten days, we will focus our energy on all different aspects of our bodies. We will look at simple changes we can make in our lives to make our bodies stronger and healthier than ever before. We will learn how to look at our bodies honestly and with love, and truly appreciate and accept what we see. We will learn to listen to our bodies and honor what they are saying to us.

Most of all, we will celebrate our bodies and how beautiful they are, in all of their different shapes and sizes. Your body is truly beautiful, right now, just the way it is. Learning to experience and celebrate that beauty is your next step in becoming a New 10.

Day 11:
I GIVE MY BODY WHAT I WANT.
I GIVE MY BODY WHAT IT NEEDS.

Beauty is eternity gazing at itself in a mirror.
— Kahlil Gibran

As women, a lot of us aren't very comfortable with our bodies. We wish they looked different, that they felt different, that they just *were* different. The thing is, we might not have such a twisted relationship with our bodies if we learned to listen to them. And learning to listen to our bodies is the first step in learning to love them.

Your body knows what it wants—and it has ways of letting you know. Getting sick is often a signal that you've been putting your body through too much and need to slow down. A headache or backache can mean we're under too much stress and need to do something calming, like meditate or take a hot bath. Tight muscles might mean that we need to stretch in a yoga or Pilates class and let those muscles really feel their strength. Feeling restless and jumpy might mean it's time to go for a walk or a run.

Our bodies don't ask much from us, but they need to be cared for to look and feel their best. All bodies need exercise and time to rejuvenate. They need to exert themselves and they need to relax. They need to work, and they need to be pampered. But the only way they can get what they need is if we care enough—and listen enough—to give it to them.

Ask yourself "do you listen to your body?" Can you read the signals it gives to you? And are you able to honor your body's physical needs? If you can learn to really honor and care for your body, you will be well on your way to becoming a New 10.

Of course, the main issue most women have with their bodies is weight, so it makes sense that the area where we most need to listen to our bodies is what we put inside them.

I don't believe in diets. And all you need to do to know they don't work is ask ten friends who have been on one! I believe the best way to control my weight—and yours too—is to think about the foods I am feeding my body.

Ask your body what it needs to operate at its highest level, and it will tell you. It needs to repair its tissues and keep its muscles strong, so it needs lean protein. It needs fresh fruits and vegetables for the vitamins, minerals, and antioxidants they provide. It needs clean whole grains for fiber, energy, and a feeling of satisfaction. It even needs some fat—healthful fats like you find in avocados, nuts, and olive oil—to stay strong and healthy and beautiful.

Feed your body what it wants, what it craves, and it will show. Your skin will glow. Excess weight will be reduced. Your brain will be sharper. You'll even sleep better! All because you listen to what your body has to say.

Of course, there will probably be times when your body seems to be asking, very plainly, for a pizza with everything on it. Or a glazed doughnut. Or a chocolate bar.

It's okay to say yes to those requests too. Everyone deserves to indulge once in awhile. If you make certain foods forbidden, chances are your brain, if not your body, will ask for them all the time, because it won't be able to stop thinking about them. The great thing is, if you concentrate on feeding your body what it *needs,* occasionally giving in to what it *wants* isn't going to hurt you.

If you do lose all control and eat an entire carton of ice cream, don't worry. Your body will probably tell you it wasn't a very good idea. And you won't do it again for a while.

Listening to your body won't always be easy. It takes some self-discipline to remember to think, to remember to ask, to remember to pay attention to the signals your body sends out. But more than anything, listening to your body is about self-love. And that's really at the core of what it means to be a New 10.

Beginning today, I want you to start really listening to your body and giving it what it needs. Remember, your body is a vessel for your spirit. How you respect that vessel determines how it will host your spirit and how your spirit can then express itself in its own beautiful way.

WHAT REALLY WORKS FOR ME

My body talks to me. And since I am a Pisces, my body often tells me it wants rich foods. It wants creamy sauces. It likes things that taste good.

Instead of ignoring my body and telling it I know better, I allow myself one day each week for those rich indulgences and one day of no calorie counting—provided they are not empty calories. This way, my body gets what it wants. And you know what? By giving my body that one day to eat whatever it craves, it craves healthful foods the other six days of the week. As I said before, it knows what it needs to stay healthy and strong.

I have been doing this for about twenty years, and given that I am the same size now as I was back then, I have to say it works.

Of course, my body also needs to move to feel toned and strong. I listen to my body there too. I exercise. My body knows when it can work harder, when it needs to rest, when to push and when to hold back. All I have to do is listen—not to impose my *own* agenda, but to respond to what my body needs each day.

Your body is the same way—it knows best what it needs. Learn to listen to it and you won't have to totally deny yourself treats. Maintaining your weight and being healthy can be delicious too!

Day 12:
I AM WEAK AND SICK.
I AM HEALTHY AND STRONG.

*The moment one gives attention to anything, even
a blade of grass, it becomes a mysterious, awesome,
indescribably magnificent world in itself.*
— Henry Miller

I can't spend a large portion of this book talking about loving our bodies without talking seriously about health. After all, the health of our bodies is linked to how we feel about our future, about ourselves, about our lives, and even about the people in our lives. So today, Day 12 of our journey, will be dedicated to taking a closer look at our health.

Getting sick is a fact of life for many women, and one we think we can't avoid. But in many cases, we can. You might not realize that your mind has tremendous power over your body. Things like stress, depression, and generally not taking care of yourself can all lead to illness. But the most damage you can do to your health comes from viewing yourself as "sick" and your body as "weak."

When we view our bodies as anything less than healthy and strong, they tend to become exactly what we see. This is partially because when we see ourselves as "sick," we treat ourselves differently and focus on different things, living a "sick person's life" instead of a "healthy person's life." Soon enough, we feel as bad as we tell ourselves we do!

If this sounds like you—if you are always suffering from some malady or other—tell yourself right now that you have the power to change that about yourself. Instead of focusing your energy on your illnesses and ailments, think about what a strong, healthy body you have. Treat your body as if it is strong and healthy; give it the right foods, exercise, and rest. Your body will reward you by becoming stronger and healthier.

Sometimes, your body will get sick just to challenge you to heal yourself. You do have that capacity. Through visualization, through concentration, through treating yourself right, you can overcome disease. An illness might represent a challenge you need to take time to overcome, or even something to change your focus to a different aspect of your life.

Of course, some of us have, or will have, health problems that are serious and real. If you are facing something like this, I believe you absolutely must see a doctor and give yourself the best care possible. Using the resources around you isn't the same thing as giving in or giving up—what you're doing is giving yourself the gift of life.

However, having a serious illness isn't a time to start viewing your body as diseased or damaged. Instead, it can be a challenge to really put the power of visualization to work for you. A health crisis is one of those things that drags you, kicking and screaming, out of your comfort zone. And like anything that pushes you beyond your normal boundaries, it offers a chance to grow and become a stronger, better, more beautiful person.

A health crisis can be an inspiration to help you focus on your health and your body. Even if you are sick, you can celebrate the parts of your body that are healthy, whatever they may be. You can focus on being healthy, on feeling healthy, on overcoming the challenges you face to live your life to the fullest, love those around you with your whole heart, and be the very best person you can be.

Whatever your personal health situation is, your body will only benefit if you spend time visualizing yourself as a vibrant, healthy, beautiful woman. Believe in your heart and soul that you can overcome any and all health challenges—and don't just talk the talk. Walk the walk and do what you need to do to keep your body healthy and strong.

Living the life that you want to live, being with the people you want to be around, and expressing your spirit as vibrantly as possible can help keep you strong through even the darkest of times.

We often take our health for granted until the moment comes when we suddenly aren't feeling so good. It's important to visualize that strong, healthy body all the time, to affirm and focus on excellent health. When you see yourself truly as a beautiful, healthy woman inside and out, you will *be* a beautiful, healthy woman inside and out. And that's the secret to becoming a New 10.

WHAT REALLY WORKS FOR ME

When you learn to listen to your body, you can hear a lot. When I really learned to tune in to the subtle signals my body sends me, I found my body actually warned me when I was about to get a cold or the flu. For me, the warning sign is when I get tired in the middle of the day and feel like I need a nap. This is not the "normal" me—I am a pretty high-energy person—so when this happens, I know it is my body telling me that something is wrong. I listen to my body and immediately switch into Prevention Mode, going to bed early and spending the next day in as low-key a way as possible, ideally just resting and relaxing and meditating.

If you listen to your body in this way, you will also learn to spot the signs of illness coming on. You will know when your body just doesn't feel right, so you will be able to take steps and do something about it before things get worse. It's an amazing thing to be able to stop a cold or flu in its tracks before it actually hits—or at least to be able to get over it in just a few days, without medication. Listening to my body has helped me take charge of my health.

It's worth getting to know your body signals this intimately. Your health and well-being need it. Good luck!

Day 13:
I SIT DOWN AND VEGETATE. I GET UP AND DANCE!

Dance as though no one is watching you, Love as though you have never been hurt before, Sing as though no one can hear you, Live as though heaven is on earth.
— Souza

As we begin our thirteenth day together and continue to focus on our beautiful bodies, I want you to take a moment and really think about your energy level. How do you feel right now, at this moment? Do you feel energetically alive?

Or do you not even know what the words *feeling energetically alive* actually mean?

In case you don't, I should probably explain. You know when your whole body feels awake and energized from head to toe—almost like you're tingling—and you feel good just about existing on this planet at this moment? That's feeling energetically alive.

Reaching this state of being means saying yes to your spirit and yes to your body. It also means that your body is physically ready for your spirit to come through and fully express itself.

If that sounds like an incredible, wonderful feeling, you're right. It is.

But if you're like a lot of women, you might feel the exact opposite of energetically alive right now. The pressures and responsibilities of day-to-day life—of your family, your friends, your job, and other issues—may be taking their toll on you. You may drag yourself out of bed in the morning, feel like you're barely surviving all day, and finally collapse in a heap at night.

When your body is exhausted, it doesn't offer your spirit much of an opportunity to express itself. In fact, when you have no energy, it tends to exhaust your spirit too.

Being exhausted with no energy is really no way to live. And it's definitely not the way to experience your true beauty.

So what can you do about it? Especially if you can't afford to take two weeks off and check in to a spa or tropical resort?

Believe it or not, there is one sure way to recapture that energy, to feel that aliveness through your whole body, and it won't cost you a thing.

All you have to do is dance. And, like the song says, to do it like no one is watching.

For the more inhibited among you, that might sound a little crazy. But I promise you, it isn't. Just put on some music that you like and start moving. You'll realize that dancing is actually simple. It's as simple as moving your hips.

And the beautiful part is, *nobody has to know you're doing it if you don't want them to.*

If you're shy and would rather crawl under a rock than let anyone see you grooving to the music, you don't have to be embarrassed. Just wait until the house is empty, put on your favorite CD or crank up your iPod, and move however your spirit tells you to.

The great thing about dance is, there is no right and wrong. It's a pure opportunity to express yourself, to express your spirit and your passion. You can dance to any type of music, from classical to heavy metal, and you can move your body in whatever way feels good and natural to you. It's all about letting your soul feel the music and express itself through your body.

If you really don't know where to start, here are a few suggestions. If you like country music, try two-stepping. Hip-hop dancing is fun and energizing. My personal favorite, belly dancing, is great because it really requires you to move your hips and get in touch with your feminine spirit.

But honestly, any kind of dance will do—ballet, tap, jazz, modern, clogging, Irish step dancing, salsa—anything at all. If you want to master some steps, you can rent a DVD or take a class. Or you can just crank up the tunes and go where the music and your body and your spirit take you.

The important thing is to get up and just do it.

You'll be amazed at how the simple act of moving to music can bring your body and spirit together and fill you with energy. You'll find you feel better all day long. You'll have more energy. Your body will benefit, and your spirit will too.

Once you've made dance a part of your everyday routine, you may also realize that—at least for you—dance is too much fun and too joyful to do in secret. So dance with your children. Dance with your husband or your boyfriend. Dance with your girlfriends.

Just move that beautiful body of yours.

And dance.

WHAT REALLY WORKS FOR ME

Everything I know about dance I owe to my daughter.

Okay, not really. I *did* dance before I became a mother—as part of that whole "other" life I had long, long ago. But part of what life as a grown-up does to you, or did to me, is that you get so busy with things you have to do, you forget about the things you love to do and need to do. In my case, I forgot what my spirit loved to do, which was dance.

This is where my daughter comes in. She has been a great teacher for me in this area, as most children are. I just watch her move with complete lack of inhibition and it inspires me to do the same. If you feel stuck, try watching children and allowing them to teach you the art of innocent expression through dance, or even singing. If you have a child, or a niece or nephew, or even a younger sibling, put on some music and dance together.

Just let your hips do the rest, and have fun!

Day 14:
I DON'T HAVE TIME TO BREATHE! I MAKE TIME TO BREATHE.

Good nature will always supply the absence of beauty;
but beauty cannot supply the absence of good nature.
— Joseph Addison

As we close out our second week of working toward becoming a New 10, I have a question for you. What if I told you there was something completely easy and effortless you could do *right now* that would improve your body and your mind?

My guess is that you would probably do it, wouldn't you?

What if I told you that something was simply to breathe?

You might think I'm not being serious.

After all, you are breathing right now, as you read this. If you weren't, you would have a real problem!

Of course, you've probably figured out that the kind of breathing I'm talking about isn't the normal, everyday, in-and-out breathing that keeps your heart pumping, your blood circulating, and your body moving. It's probably not the kind of breathing you're doing right now. Not that that kind isn't important.

I'm talking about an entirely different kind of breathing—focused, intentional, deep breathing that quiets your mind, helps you relax, helps you focus and center and ground yourself. This kind of breathing is very similar to meditation. In fact, it actually *is* meditation. But don't let the word scare you off. Although the idea of *meditation* might conjure up images of wise religious men sitting cross-legged on mountaintops, the reality is very different.

Meditation is, at its core, very simple, basic breathing. It's about taking the time to find a moment of quiet, even if it's just for a few minutes, a few times a day, to experience your breath, which is your life force and a true gift from God. If you can make this small time commitment for yourself every day, the results can actually be life changing. You will feel centered and grounded with each breath that you take, and you will be flooded with positive feelings and energy that will help you feel better about yourself both physically and mentally.

By taking this quiet time to simply breathe, we let go of the cares of the day. We silence the voices in our heads. And we open that space inside of us to the divine guidance of the universe. When we stop and simply breathe, the answers we need that we might miss because we're too busy with our day-to-day lives have a chance to come to us.

How do we accomplish this type of breathing? Find a quiet spot right now, take the phone off the hook, and I will talk you through an exercise.

Sit down in a way that is comfortable for you. You can try the lotus position or a half lotus, or simply sit on the floor with your legs crossed. Try to sit up as straight as you can. If you have trouble, you can even balance yourself against a wall or on a chair, but the idea is to be as upright as possible so you can really fill your lungs with air.

Now close your eyes—actually, you should close them after you're finished reading this part—and breathe in as slowly and deeply as you can. Concentrate on your breathing. It might help to slowly count to five as you breathe in to keep your mind focused only on the breath you are taking. Feel your lungs filling with air and your rib cage expanding and your spirit filling with light. Once your lungs are completely filled, let the air out just as slowly, to the count of five. Again, concentrate on the feeling of the air leaving your lungs.

Repeat this for at least ten breaths, at least three times a day, to notice results.

Once you've mastered this breathing technique, you can even add a little visualization to make a difference on an energetic and cellular level. For example, if you want to feel love or bring more love into your life, close your eyes and imagine you are bringing in pink light as you breathe. You can see it when you close your eyes if you really concentrate. If you want to feel empowered, try doing the same with blue light. If you are not feeling well or have suffered an injury, breathe in green light and feel it reaching deep into your cells and healing them with each breath.

The fact is, you can breathe in whatever color makes you feel the way you want to feel, whatever color is significant to you. Just close your eyes and breathe deeply and feel the light filling you and washing over you. If you do this every day, I promise that you will feel a difference almost immediately. You will feel more centered, more energized, and even more beautiful.

And you'll be ready to tackle the next step in our journey.

WHAT REALLY WORKS FOR ME

When I first started concentrating on my breathing, I was shocked to discover that my natural breathing pattern was really shallow. This affected my stress levels—all that fast, shallow breathing kept me from fully relaxing. It also prevented me from experiencing the full strength of my intuitive powers.

What works for me is simply reminding myself and doing it, every single day. At first, I left myself notes around the house—on the bathroom mirror, on my pillow, on the refrigerator—that simply said "Breathe!" Those reminders taught me to pay attention to my breath at each moment I spotted them. Often I would stop right then and take my ten deep breaths, until I began doing it at more regular times each day.

Learning to breathe properly and fully taught me that my breath is truly a gift from God. Breathing purposefully has helped me become more heart centered and calmer.

There are many different types of breathing exercises, and I recommend that you do what feels right to you. Try to breathe deeply for at least ten breaths and do it three times a day. It's easy to remember if you do it in the morning, in midafternoon, and before you go to bed. Just get into a routine, and it will become part of your life. All it takes is a couple of minutes ... and, yes, you're worth it!

Day 15:
I DON'T NEED VITAMINS. I NEED VITAMINS, MINERALS, AND ANTIOXIDANTS.

It matters more what's in a women's face than what's on it.
— Claudette Colbert

Today is Day 15 of our journey together, and we'll begin our third week by continuing our focus on our beautiful bodies. I want to take this day to talk about something you've probably been hearing all your life, from your parents when you were a child to your doctor today:

Take your vitamins!

(Not only that, but to keep your body feeling good from the inside out, you also need to take your minerals and antioxidants.)

Why? Well, as we women get older, it becomes more and more important to honor the vitamin needs of our bodies to keep them strong and healthy. Although you may eat all the right foods, exercise, and do everything you should to maintain your body, supplements are in many cases the only way your body can possibly get enough of what it needs to operate at its peak and avoid disease and other problems in the future.

According to experts, there are eleven essential vitamins and minerals that you need every day to stay healthy.

Vitamin A is important to your eyes and skin. It's difficult to get enough simply from your diet, so a supplement is probably a good idea. However, most multivitamins actually contain too much of it if you have a healthful diet, so look with one that contains only 50 percent of your daily value. A good alternative is beta-carotene, which is also an essential and converts to vitamin A in the body.

The B vitamins, which ensure health cell growth, are plentiful in foods like breads and cereals, so unless you are deficient, you should not need to supplement your intake of B6, B12, riboflavin, thiamin, and niacin. If your diet is lacking, however, err on the side of caution and take a supplement.

You will definitely want to add to your intake of vitamin C, even if you drink a lot of orange juice and get a lot in your diet. Vitamin C is a powerful antioxidant and immune system booster, and it also fights free radicals that hurt our bodies and dull our skin.

The same goes for folic acid, which helps your body form red and white blood cells and helps prevent birth defects in pregnant women.

Vitamin E has amazing powers to keep you beautiful on the outside while taking care of your insides, so your multivitamin should contain some E.

Women tend to be low in iron, so a supplement is a good idea here. However, in this case you must be careful not to take too much, as iron can be toxic at high levels.

You may not have heard of vitamin K, but it works with vitamin D and calcium to build your bones, so it's an essential for women, especially as we grow older.

That goes double for vitamin D: your body can't absorb calcium without it, so you absolutely must make sure you get enough of it every day.

Of course, when it comes to things women need, the mineral calcium tops the list. Not getting enough calcium can lead to bone loss and osteoporosis in a frighteningly large percentage of women, so if you add only one thing in this chapter to your daily routine, it should be calcium (with some vitamin D and vitamin K thrown in to aid absorption, of course!). If you take calcium every day in your multivitamin, you should take a separate calcium supplement again at another point in the day. As much as your body needs this precious mineral, it can absorb only less than half of what you need in a day at a time.

Finally, the mineral magnesium, which protects against heart disease, colon cancer, and diabetes, is another essential that is often left out of basic multivitamins, so make sure to read the label before you buy.

Beyond these essentials, there are other health supplements on the market that could be beneficial to your overall health, depending on your diet and your individual needs. They range from omega-3 fatty acids to garlic supplements to seaweed, and many, many more I don't have room to list here.

The best way to find out what your needs are—and a good idea in general since you are going to take better care of your beautiful body from now on!—is to see your doctor or health professional. Talk together about what supplements you might need to keep your body in top form. You may notice a change almost immediately, in your inner strength and inner beauty, as well as your energy level, your hair, skin, and nails, and in the overall way you feel about yourself. After all, a healthy body is a beautiful body.

And that's the kind of body you deserve.

WHAT REALLY WORKS FOR ME

Basically, it comes down to training myself to make vitamins and other supplements a part of my routine. I take my vitamins every morning—it's as much a part of my morning ritual as taking a shower or brushing my teeth. I just make it an automatic part of my day so I never forget.

I also really like a product called Borba. It is an antioxidant powder that you mix with water and drink daily. I take it once a day along with my vitamins and other supplements. It helps cut down the yeast level in my body, which makes my skin look amazing. I look at it as skin care from the inside out.

You can learn more about Borba and order it at www.borba.com. I hope you like it as much as I do!

Day 16:
MY CORE IS WEAK.
MY CORE IS STRONG.

Everything you need is already inside. Just do it.
— Bill Bowerman (cofounder of Nike)

As we continue talking about our physical bodies, I'd like to take a look at your inner strength. As we get older, many of us feel that strength—our physical inner strength—slipping away. We feel pain where we once felt fine, are less flexible, and generally sense that our bodies are no longer in their prime. That is, if they were ever in their prime in the first place.

Many women think this is a natural part of the aging process. And although it is true and natural that we will all lose some of our physical capacity as we age, I am here to tell you that you can look and feel amazing right now, whatever your age.

I am a forty-five-year-old woman and I've given birth to three children. I've also been through three major abdominal surgeries. But despite my age and the wear and tear on my stomach muscles, my tummy is still flat. I still have a trim, slim waist. And my body is strong. The reason? I have developed and maintain a strong core.

Your core muscles are really the core of your physical body. They're the muscles of your stomach and middle and lower back. When they are powerful and strong, they keep you not only slim but healthy. They help you to stand and sit up straight, and take pressure off other parts of your body, which really cuts down on aches and pains.

Of course, if you haven't been exercising regularly, chances are your core may not be particularly strong. Maybe your body isn't in the best of shape. Believe it or not, it is never too late to change this, and it can be done fairly simply. My advice to you and all women out there—and my own secret to staying strong and in shape—is to try Pilates or power yoga.

Both of these exercise techniques focus on strengthening your core, with an additional emphasis on deep breathing techniques, which are strengthening and relaxing, and balance. Both start at the beginner level and allow you to work at your own pace, beginning with simple stretches and poses and moving into more difficult moves as you become stronger and more flexible.

Pilates can be performed in two different ways. The original form of Pilates is done with the help of a trainer or instructor on an apparatus called a Reformer—a machine specifically designed to work your core muscles. The benefits of this form of Pilates are tremendous. Each workout is specifically tailored to you and your fitness level, from an absolute beginner in very weak physical shape to a seasoned athlete. With a trainer guiding you at all times, you will work your body in a way that feels comfortable but is also tremendously effective for you.

The downside, however, is that an hour on the Reformer with your own trainer can be expensive.

Mat Pilates and power yoga are far more affordable alternatives. These are Pilates or yoga poses, moves and exercises, breathing and balance techniques designed to be performed either with nothing but a mat or with simple, inexpensive equipment like balls or stretch bands.

You can do Pilates or yoga in a class, which is probably the best choice for those who have not exercised in a while, as it's helpful to have professional guidance when you start out. Just sign up for a beginner's class—just about every town has at least one—and let your instructor know upfront what your limitations are. He or she will work with you to grow your core strength over time.

If the thought of going to a gym or class terrifies you, you can still learn some of these techniques through books or videos. However, I really encourage you to let a professional guide you if you are not in shape, at least when you start out. A professional can teach you the best techniques to help you with your specific needs, and also make sure that you do the right moves in the right way so you don't injure yourself. After all, strengthening your core is about making you feel better, not worse!

Once you begin working your core, amazing things will begin to happen, no matter what kind of shape you're in to begin with. Your back will become strengthened and you'll feel less pain. You'll stand taller. Your flexibility will increase. And perhaps most important, increased physical strength will give you more energy—energy that will make you stronger, more alive, and more beautiful, no matter how old you are.

WHAT REALLY WORKS FOR ME

For me, the perfect place to work out is at home. I realize this might not work for you; some people prefer a gym and some people just don't have the space to stretch out at home. But for me, not having to leave the house and drive somewhere and having the flexibility to work out when I want to makes it easy to get my workouts in. I have worked out at least four or five days per week for the past twenty-five years this way, so it definitely works for me.

Especially after having children, the most important thing to develop has been my core strength. It's been more effective than aerobics. I like a DVD put out by The Firm called *Power Yoga*; you can find it on amazon.com. It offers great core strengthening exercises as well as strength and flexibility exercises.

Working with a balance ball is also effective for core strengthening, and I use it at least three times a week.

I highly recommend that you try any core-strengthening program and give it a good month trial. You will feel so much better that you won't want to stop!

Day 17:
I HIDE FROM MY SEXUALITY.
I EMBRACE MY SEXUALITY.

Sex and beauty are inseparable, like life and consciousness. And the intelligence which goes with sex and beauty, and arises out of sex and beauty, is intuition.
— D. H. Lawrence

Today is going to be a very important day on our journey. We've spent sixteen days together. Ideally we've gotten to know each other a little over this time, and ideally we've gotten a little more comfortable trying new things and looking at ourselves in a new way. So now, on Day 17, while we're still on the subject of our bodies, I think we're finally ready to tackle one of the hardest subjects to talk about.

I'm talking, of course, about our sexuality.

Sexuality shouldn't be that difficult to discuss. After all, our sexuality is a natural part of us. It's part of what makes us divine, what makes us feminine. It's a gift from God, and it's meant to be celebrated and enjoyed.

But unfortunately, for some of us, talking about sex is easier said— or in this case written about—than done. For whatever reason, many of us just don't feel safe in our sexuality. Maybe we've been conditioned to think that having sexual urges and feelings is wrong, that "nice girls" don't feel those things, so we don't feel comfortable expressing that part of ourselves. Instead, we stuff our sexual feelings and needs down inside, or deny ourselves true enjoyment in this area instead of celebrating something that is our divine right as women.

Maybe you are one of many, many women who have a healthy relationship with their sexuality. Maybe you are able to fully enjoy a satisfying sex life where you can express yourself freely. For all of you who can experience this freedom right now, I congratulate you and urge you to keep it up. Part of experiencing the full power of your beauty—both inside and outside—is expressing your beauty through a healthy sex life, so it's wonderful that you already have that power.

But for those of us who don't fit into the group I just talked about, feeling safe in your sexuality can be a real challenge. It can be hard to feel comfortable expressing that part of yourself, either alone or in relationships. And maybe, if you're one of those people who have settled for a less-than-stellar sex life, you have decided that this is the most comfortable place for you to be and a place where you are destined to stay.

If that's the case, I want you to remember what I said a few days ago about expanding your comfort zone. If sexuality is currently not a part of yours, you need to stretch your comfort zone just a little and allow some sexuality in.

I realize this is a difficult area for a lot of women. But it's also really, really important to fully experiencing your true beauty as a woman, both inside and out. Remember, when you cut off a part of yourself or stifle a part of yourself, it can't bloom or grow, so it can't add that extra dimension to your beauty. But when you let those parts of yourself into the light, your true beauty shines through.

Sex, especially with someone you love, can be a spiritual experience, uniting your mind, your body, and your soul. It is a natural process that can be a very beautiful thing. It makes you feel good, and it makes you feel beautiful, and it can foster your spirit in many, many ways. That means sexuality is more than natural and healthy. Truly experiencing and feeling comfortable with your sexuality is an important step toward reaching your full potential as a New 10.

That's not to say that dealing with your sexuality is always going to be easy, especially at first. I have my challenges in this area too. But it really does serve us to learn to honor our sexuality …fully express our sexuality and …fully enjoy our sexuality. It's all part of the divine, and it's all a gift from God. It's here to enrich your life and make it beautiful.

And a beautiful life is something we all deserve.

WHAT REALLY WORKS FOR ME

To be honest, meeting the right partner was really the key to my sexual bliss. Having the right person to share my sexuality with makes the experience that much more beautiful—and more fun!

But I can say that getting more in touch with my sexuality helped draw this person into my life, and has helped me more fully enjoy our time together. Whether you have found Mr. Right or are still looking, it is never too early to encourage yourself to grow in this area, even if you're not entirely comfortable with it!

Growing as a woman, getting more in touch with my spirituality, and embracing my divine feminine nature really helped my sexuality blossom. I didn't look at my sexuality in a vacuum, I saw it as part of the whole package that made me. So as I grew, it grew. Embrace the beautiful woman you are, body and soul, and you will free yourself to enjoy your sexuality more than you ever have.

I also do some energy work and chakra balancing to help wake up my kundalini energy. ... The higher my vibration, the greater the experience.

Just remember, you are infinitely beautiful and perfect, just as you are, so enjoy yourself!

Day 18:
I AM A MESS.
I AM PERFECT.

I said to myself—I'll paint what I see—what the flower is to me but I'll paint it big and they will be surprised into tasking time to look at it—I will make even busy New Yorkers take time to see what I see of flowers.
— Georgia O'Keeffe

Welcome back to our journey to experiencing your true beauty together. It's now Day 18, and time to tackle another question that might be a little difficult for you.

Can you honestly stand in front of a mirror and feel beautiful regardless of what you see? Even with your clothes off?

Or do you pick yourself apart from head to toe? Do you focus on every little flaw, every lump and line and bulge, to the point where you can't even see the overall picture of who you are, only a collection of things that "need fixing"?

If the second answer sounds like you, you are not alone. This chapter is for you and everyone like you. Because as women, we have some serious work to do!

With the messages that society gives us, with size zero models smiling perfect smiles at us from the pages of magazines, it's easy to fall into the trap of believing we just don't measure up. But as women, we need to avoid that trap at all costs. We need to look in the mirror and love and accept what we see, flaws and all. We need to accept who we are as beautiful.

Does this mean we can't work toward changing parts of ourselves to make them better? Absolutely not. There are some parts of our bodies that we can change. We can exercise or choose more healthful foods to change our body shape, or to give our bodies more strength and more energy. We can change the color or style of our hair, wear makeup to accentuate or hide our features, and more.

But as you probably know, this can be a slippery slope. The line between the woman who erases a few frown lines with some Botox injections and the woman with a motionless, unlined, and unnatural face gets thinner all the time. There are women—and even some men—who feel compelled to remake every aspect of their bodies and faces through plastic surgery. There are even women who go under the knife trying to look like a specific celebrity or a Barbie doll.

Obviously, a woman who will do this to her body—put it through this kind of torture and spend tens of thousands of dollars to do it—does not love what she sees in the mirror. A woman who is constantly grasping at medical "solutions" to her appearance can never find her true beauty, because she can never be her true self.

That's why it is so, so important to find that level of acceptance and love for the woman you are right now. Yes, you can work to be the very best you can be. But the key is to be the best version of *you* that you can be and not to be someone else. You are beautiful right now, the way you are. Any changes you make should enhance and celebrate that beauty, not destroy everything what you are already.

This attitude becomes more important when we deal with other aspects of our physical bodies that we don't have the power to change. Your body is a certain type, a certain shape. You have a genetic history that makes you *you,* and at some point you need to accept it and love it. Your eyes are going to be the color they are, your skin the color it is, and your hair has a certain texture. You may not be able to change those things dramatically. But you shouldn't feel the need to. Your hair, your eyes, and your skin are all the things that make you *you.* And they are the things that make you beautiful, not looking like a cookie-cutter copy of a woman in a magazine.

I believe that on some level, we all agreed to come into this lifetime with the bodies we have right now. I feel we chose our bodies for a reason, and it really serves us to accept our bodies as beautiful regardless of how they work or look.

The truth is, even if you are trying to make a physical change, these changes don't always come about very easily, especially without the serene acceptance of who we are right now. Without acceptance we actually spend more time beating ourselves up for what we're not than working in a positive way toward what we want to be.

I want you to spend some time actually looking at yourself in the mirror and seeing how beautiful you are—because you are. We are all intrinsically beautiful.

Remember that, and your beauty will only grow.

WHAT REALLY WORKS FOR ME

As a child, I was repeatedly told that I was ugly and fat, so feeling beautiful was something that did not happen for me until I was past forty. It's still a work in progress.

For me, loving what I see means taking care of myself so that I am the best I can be.

I go to professional salons to get my hair done. I use high-quality products on my hair, skin, and body. And yes, I even use Botox and fillers. Some of you might be surprised to hear that. For me, it's not about changing my physical appearance but about maintaining it. I don't want to be someone else; I want to be the best *me* I can be.

That said, I'm a normal woman. Some days I feel better than others about my body. On the not-so-good days, I remind myself to be that much more grateful for my body instead of looking for faults with it. I think about all the good that my body does for me, and it gets me through the rough times.

I recommend from experience that instead of comparing yourself with anyone else, you instead look at your body as a unique, beautiful vessel for your spirit that was chosen by you, for you, and to serve you. Then extend a big thank-you to God for that gift. You are that beautiful!

Day 19:
I HIDE MY BODY.
I FLAUNT MY BODY.

Sex appeal is fifty percent what you've got and fifty percent what people think you've got.
— Sophia Loren

Welcome to another day on our journey together. Over the past few days, as we've really zeroed in on our bodies, I hope you've found new ways to accept, strengthen, and appreciate your body and the wonder that it is. And yes, I do mean flaws and all, because your flaws are part of what makes you unique and what makes you *you*.

But today, we're not focusing on our flaws. Today, we're going to take our exploration of our bodies one step further. We're going to celebrate our bodies by finding and focusing on the one part of our physical selves that makes us feel the best about ourselves. You're going to find that part of your body you just know is fabulous—whatever it might be—and you're going to flaunt it.

Do you flaunt the fabulous in you? A lot of women don't. If you've ever seen a makeover show on TV or a feature on makeovers in a magazine, you know many of us tend to overlook our best features.

Some women hide great figures under baggy clothes, or leave beautiful faces without makeup, and just generally hide their gifts from the world.

Why? There are many different reasons. Some women feel uncomfortable calling attention to themselves, as if asking for attention is somehow wrong. Others spend so much time focusing on things they don't like about themselves that they actually forget about the good parts. And other women get so bogged down in their day-to-day lives that they stop taking the time to see themselves as desirable, feminine, and beautiful.

But you are beautiful. And today is all about putting you back in touch with that part of yourself.

The first step is to take a good look at yourself from head to toe. Don't forget your backside too. Look yourself over with loving eyes, and find that one part of yourself you just know is fabulous. Maybe you have an amazing head of hair. Or beautiful, expressive eyes. Maybe you have shapely shoulders, or fabulous ankles, or sexy legs, or lovely feet. Everyone has something, and you are no exception. That's your first assignment. Look in the mirror and find that fabulous feature that you are proud of.

Found it? Great. Now I want you to take that body part, whatever it is, and find a way to flaunt it—every day. Flaunt it as often as you want, in as many ways as you can imagine.

How do you flaunt your best feature? Obviously it depends on what that feature is, but here are a few ideas. If your best feature is your eyes, try wearing colors that make those beautiful eyes pop. If you have great hair, keep it shiny and well conditioned to show it off. If your best feature is your figure, wear a short skirt to spotlight gorgeous legs, or a racer-back top to showcase your shoulders, or a low-cut blouse to flash just a little cleavage. Paint your toenails in your favorite color and buy strappy sandals to focus on your fabulous feet.

The important thing isn't what your specific body part is. The idea here is to find a way, or even several ways, to flaunt it and celebrate it. Those parts of you that are fabulous are your special gifts from God. We all possess some amazing, beautiful feature, and whatever it is for you, it's time for you to celebrate it and flaunt it and show it off to anyone and everyone you run across. It's yours, you own it, and most of all, you deserve it.

When you focus on the part of you that makes you feel good about yourself, that good feeling is infectious. When you showcase the beauty of just one part, that good feeling radiates through you and helps you feel beautiful all over. And as you continue to flaunt your one favorite part, you may find other areas that also catch your eye, and you'll start flaunting those too, until you are celebrating and flaunting your unique, individual beauty as a woman.

It may sound like a lot, but remember, it all starts simply, with one small body part. If you flaunt that fabulous part of yourself today, you'll start to not only feel beautiful from the inside out but to show that beauty to the world.

And that's what being a New 10 is all about.

WHAT REALLY WORKS FOR ME

Turning forty was a pivotal point in my life. It was the point where I decided to stop trying to look how I was "supposed" to and look how I wanted to. That meant giving up the conservative, baggy "mom" look and switching to a more sophisticated, sexy look. I have never felt more like myself than when I started wearing the fabrics I loved next to my skin and wearing the colors I loved. It also felt good to celebrate my body in clothes that didn't hide my curves from the world.

There's nothing I love more than bit of "bling," and I dress accordingly—some might say a little *too* accordingly. But I'm not dressing for other people anymore. I'm dressing for *me*. And the feminine goddess inside of me loves nothing more than to sparkle and shine.

What does your inner goddess want to wear? Silky fabrics that flow? Bright colors? Or her own bit of bling? Whatever it is, dress your goddess the way she wants to dress, and your true beauty can't help but shine through.

Day 20
I HAVE AN UGLY SMILE.
I HAVE A BEAUTIFUL SMILE.

Joy is the best makeup.
— Anne Lamotte

Wow. Today marks the halfway point of our journey together. It's Day 20, and time to wind up our focus on our physical bodies and move on to other aspects of beauty. I want to finish this section in a powerful way, with what I think might be the most powerful, important thing you can do with your body. The best news is, it also happens to be one of the easiest.

I want you to smile.

We all look better when we smile. Even if our teeth are less than perfect, it doesn't matter. Honestly, there's nothing more captivating than a real, genuine smile. When we smile, our true beauty shines through. We radiate our energy to the world and everyone around us. We show that we are open and friendly and positive.

But that's not all smiling can do for you. It also has a secret power.

When you smile, you actually feel happier.

The simple act of smiling can change your state of feeling and your state of being. Don't believe me? Try it. Right now, in the middle of reading this, just stop and smile.

Maybe you felt a little silly, sitting there grinning at a page in a book—which is good! It probably gave you something to smile at.

But along with the silliness, did you also feel a little spark of happiness?

Ideally you did. It is almost impossible to feel bad while smiling. But it's not completely impossible. If you're feeling especially depressed or low, the simple act of smiling might not be enough to get you there.

Luckily, I have a trick for you too. If you didn't feel anything the first time you smiled, if there was no spark of happiness whatsoever, I want you to try it again. But this time, I want you to try to think of something happy while you smile. Think of the face of someone you love, smiling at you. Think of something that made you laugh, even if it was only in a movie or on TV. Look outside if it's a beautiful day and think about what a beautiful world we live in.

No matter what kind of a day you're having, no matter what may be going on in your life, I promise you there is always something, somewhere to feel happy about. And there is always a reason to smile.

How often do you smile? Think about it. Do you smile at strangers in the supermarket or walking down the street? Do you smile at all like you just did, when you're all alone and no one is looking? Can you see the humorous side of life, or the beauty in life, or the joy in life, and just let yourself smile at the world around you and the people in it?

I have certainly not been perfect in this area. For a long time, I didn't smile enough. I was bogged down with the challenges of work, parenthood, and getting through my day-to-day existence. But once I realized how little I smiled, I started really thinking about it. I reminded myself to smile at people when I was out running errands. I reminded myself to think of the good things in my life throughout the day—things that made me smile.

And you know what? The more I smiled, the better I felt. The better I felt, the more I smiled. Pretty soon I was smiling almost all the time.

It can work that way for you too. In fact, smiling is contagious: the more you smile, the more people will smile back at you. In a small way, just by smiling, you'll be making the world a better place. You'll be bringing a tiny moment of happiness to the people you encounter, every single time you smile at them. Ideally they will pass it on to the people they encounter. And all that joy will have come from you.

What can be more beautiful than that?

WHAT REALLY WORKS FOR ME

I strive to constantly create my life in accordance with the guidance of my soul and the desires of my heart. In other words, I try to do the things that make me feel happy. I try to live in such a way that my life is filled with joy. By living a happy, fulfilling life most of the time, I find that I can't help smiling, because I have so much to smile about.

But even on a bad day, when I don't feel quite so "smiley," all I need to do is pause and think for a moment. I remind myself that, even on a bad day, I am living authentically. I am empowering myself to live transparently and on purpose.

What is your soul guiding you to do or be?

What is your heart urging to do or be?

When you hear its messages, act on it. ... You will have much to smile about if you do!

I IGNORE MY SPIRIT.
I EMBRACE MY SPIRIT.

I would rather be a superb meteor, every atom of me in magnificent glow, than a sleepy and permanent planet. The proper function of a man is to live, not to exist.
— Jack London

Our beauty may start in our minds, and it may show itself to the world in the form of our bodies, but there is one place where our beauty is more powerful than any other. And that is within our spirit.

Our spirit is where our hearts and souls express themselves in their purest form. It is the part of us where everything is honest and good and beautiful. In fact, it is where true beauty comes from. You've probably never heard of anyone having an "ugly spirit," because there simply is no such thing. When we access our spirits, and we express ourselves through our spirits, our true beauty shines through.

Of course, most of us are caught up in the day-to-day, decidedly nonspiritual business of life. We have so much to do, so much to accomplish during the day, that it can be difficult to take time out and focus on our spirits.

And to be honest, many of us wouldn't know where to begin in the first place.

We know our spirits are there and that they are important, but we aren't exactly sure what to do with them!

So I am dedicating the third part of this book to our beautiful spirits.

Together, we will spend the next ten days focusing on this often overlooked part of ourselves. We'll learn how to listen to them. How to honor them. And most important, how to express them.

When we live through our spirits, when we let our spirits take the lead, our true beauty can really shine through. That kind of beauty—that beauty that comes from the spirit—is probably the biggest part of becoming a New 10.

So read on ... and get ready to shine.

Day 21:
I FEAR THE UNIVERSE.
I TRUST THE UNIVERSE.

I am bigger than anything that can happen to me. All these things, sorrow, misfortune, and suffering, are outside my door. I am in the house and I have the key.
— Charles Fletcher Lummis

Hello and welcome to Day 21! I hope that today, as we reach the milestone of three whole weeks together, you are feeling more beautiful than ever before, both inside and out. Ideally each day, you have gotten to know the incredible, amazing woman you truly are a little better, and are learning how to celebrate her and let her be the very best she can be. I especially hope you're feeling ready for the second half of our journey to becoming a New 10, because that second half begins today.

As we move past our minds and our bodies and on to the larger area of our spirits, I'd first like you to take a look at your place in the universe. Do you feel that you have one? And do you trust the universe to give you what you need, no matter what?

Trusting the universe can be a tricky proposition, especially if when I say the word *universe,* you picture stars and planets and something like a scene out of a science fiction movie. Yes, the physical universe, where the Milky Way and the solar system and all those things are, is certainly part of the universe I'm talking about. But there is much more to it than that.

When I refer to the universe, I'm really talking about God and about the divine, although I understand that this concept means different things to different people. I'm referring to the force that has power over our lives. I'm referring to this beautiful world, and the people in it, and everyone and everything around you. The universe is infinite and powerful. But despite how all-encompassing it is, you are still a very important part of it.

It's hard for a lot of people to see themselves connected to the universe simply because it is so big, and we are so very, very small in comparison. But the truth is, we are all profoundly connected to the universe. Everything we do affects the universe in some way, however small. And of course, the universe affects us as well.

Whatever we do and wherever we go, the universe has a say. Sometimes when something goes wrong, ranging from an occasion when we don't get something we want to something that is actually tragic, horrible, and painful, it happens because the universe wants it to be that way. Even because it *has* to be that way.

This is where the whole idea of trusting the universe comes into play. If you've been through a lot of pain in your life, you may feel like the universe is harsh and cruel. It can be difficult to see the universe as benevolent, or see that it is really conspiring for your good.

We've all heard the expression "Things happen for a reason." And it's true. Just because you can't see or understand the reason for something going wrong doesn't mean there isn't one. If we can learn to trust that we will get through the hard times, if we can put our trust in the universe, or in God, we can open ourselves up to the wonderful, magical things that the universe actually has in store for us.

When we experience problems or issues, trusting that a friendly universe is guiding us can teach us to view them as opportunities. And when we just let go and trust in the universe, we open up a gateway of miracles and synchronicities that happen without our even trying.

Please understand, it's not about completely letting go of everything. We're still going to have real emotions and reactions when things go wrong. But if we can just meet the universe halfway—if we can simply acknowledge that it is there, that it is good, and that it is looking out for us—this magical change can begin.

I have learned about this firsthand. I lost a baby girl. She was stillborn, and the pain was unbelievable. But later, when I pushed through the pain of childbirth to meet my son, who I later lost in an open adoption process, I was finally able to see and trust in the workings of the universe and that it wasn't conspiring to hurt me or to make my life miserable. My son was born twelve weeks prematurely and had only a five percent survival rate. Against all odds, he lived only for me to lose him later through the adoption process. Yes, I had a broken heart, but I was able to heal it. And along the way I learned to love more openly, more clearly, more courageously, and more wisely.

There's always a gift in our tragedies. The universe makes sure of it. Our job is simply to trust that it's there.

WHAT REALLY WORKS FOR ME

I have made a conscious choice to view the universe, with all its power and glory, as very friendly. I really believe that God wants us to be happy.

I know that trusting in a benevolent universe works because I have been there. I lost two children, and I experienced an almost unbelievable amount of pain and grief in the process. But the pain did not destroy me. It deepened me. It changed me. It helped me grow. And it actually became the gateway to my experiencing an authentic love, joy, and reverence for life.

If I believe my life is a journey, which I do, then everything that happens to me, both good and bad, is a necessary part of the journey. To me, this means that even the bad things can't actually be classified as "bad," because they are all part of making me the person I need to be, of helping me grow and reach my full potential. If it is my calling to help others—something I believe to be true—I wouldn't be much good if I had an easy, painless life free of challenges. How could I relate to other people's pain if I did not know what pain felt like?

I have made a conscious choice to heal and truly live my life to full capacity, because I know that a rich, full life is what the universe wants for me.

I did it, and I know that you can too!

Day 22:
I HAVE A SOUL?
I HAVE A SOUL!

*Meditate. Live purely. Be quiet. Do your work with mastery.
Like the moon, come out from behind the clouds! Shine.*
— Buddha

As we continue exploring our spiritual sides, I'm going to ask you a fairly unusual question (although you might be getting used to some of those by now!). The subject for Day 22 on our journey is the soul—our relationship with our soul and our connection to our soul. My question for you is, How well do you know your soul? Do you know her favorite colors, the fragrances she loves, her favorite music, her favorite sounds? Are you that intimate with your soul that you can actually speak for her?

"Of course," you might be saying. "Isn't my soul *me*? Wouldn't everything my soul likes be identical to what *I* like?"

The answer is, not necessarily.

Your soul is you. In fact, your soul is the deepest, truest, most complete expression of you and who you are. But that *you* isn't always the *you* you take out in the regular, everyday world. It isn't the face you always show to strangers, or at the office, or to friends and family, or even to yourself. In fact, depending on how well you know yourself and how closely you listen to yourself, you may not really know your soul very well at all.

Let me try an example. Let's think about music. Say all your friends listen to country music, so you do too. You buy country albums. You've programmed all the buttons on your car radio to country stations. Your iPod is loaded with country tunes. As far as you're concerned, you're a country-music lover.

Now say you go out to dinner to a nice restaurant where jazz is playing in the background. You've never really listened to jazz before; it's not on your car radio, it's not on your iPod, your friends don't like it. You can't name a single jazz song or artist. (Except maybe Frank Sinatra, but everyone knows him!) But as you sit in the restaurant listening to the music, you feel yourself being transported. You can't explain it, but something about the music touches you.

That's your soul. And apparently, it really likes jazz.

Please understand, I am in no way saying that country music is bad for your soul or that you need to go out and buy some jazz albums immediately. I'm just encouraging you to become aware of what touches *your* soul. It's different for every person, but it may not be what you expect it to be.

Some people can actually physically feel when something reaches so deeply inside them that it touches their soul. They may get emotional or teary, or they may briefly feel a flush or a tingle. Souls like these are very sensitive and expressive, and if you have one, it's probably much easier to know and understand what your soul likes.

If you're not as in touch with your soul, don't worry. There are real, practical things you can do to connect with your soul. For me, a powerful channel has been my dreams. Before I go to bed, I ask my soul to come to me in my dreams and share information with me about what she loves and what she needs from me. Then, first thing in the morning,

I jot down everything I remember from the night before. This is a really simple way to get to know your soul.

If you don't remember your dreams when you wake up in the morning, that's okay. You can also call your soul to you before you get out of bed. Ask her to be with you all day to guide you, to guide everything you do, everything you say, all your movements, all your interactions. You know what? Once you start listening to your soul, and considering what she wants for herself and for you, you'll start to know your soul inside and out.

Getting in touch with your soul can be life changing, because when you do, you get in touch with the most true, most honest, and most beautiful part of yourself. The better you know your soul—and the more you express what is in your soul in your everyday life—the more beautiful you will be. Becoming one with your soul means you will operate through that most beautiful part of you all the time. That is why your relationship with your soul is probably the most important relationship you're going to have in your life.

Get to know her, listen to her, and most of all, let her guide you. The more you do, the more your beauty will grow. And that's what being a New 10 is all about: radiating from your beautiful soul.

WHAT REALLY WORKS FOR ME

Meditation has proved to be the most surefire way for me to get in touch with my soul. When I am in complete quiet, focused only on my breathing, my soul speaks to me, and I can speak to her and ask her what she wants, how she feels, what she needs. I know *I* need this special time, away from ringing phones and an inbox full of e-mails and a daughter who needs to be driven to a friend's house, to stay connected to who I really am.

This is why I *love* Orin's meditations and programs and why I work with all of them. Instead of tackling the idea of meditation and trying to get in touch with my soul on my own, these guided meditations gave me the tools to help me get where I needed to go. Orin led me to my first experience in knowing my soul, and I have grown with her daily since I started doing the programs seven years ago.

Of course, this is not the only path to knowing your own soul, I only know how much it has done for me. If this path is of interest to you, I guarantee it is a gentle and loving approach to growing as your soul and as your divine self. You can learn more about Orin's programs at www.orindaben.com.

You are a beautiful soul. ... It is your divine right to know her and express her!

Day 23:

I AM POWERLESS.
I AM POWERFUL.

Love all. Serve all. Help ever. Hurt never.
— Author Unknown

As we talk more about our spirits and our souls, and get to know and understand our divine beauty and our divine selves better, you may actually be able to feel yourself changing as you grow closer and closer to becoming that New 10 woman. And as you do, you might be noticing something surprising about yourself. You may be feeling more powerful than you have in the past.

I'm not talking about physical strength, although if you've been trying some of the tips in the last section of this book and really honoring and celebrating your body, your body may very well be growing stronger by the day.

Right now, I'm talking about a different kind of power. Your divine power.

You may not know what divine power is, let alone know that you have it. But trust me, you do. All women do. It's part of what makes us women. It's part of what lies inside our spirits and our souls. As we work through the chapters of this book—as we express our spirits and souls and our needs and desires more frequently, more fluently, and more freely—we unleash that divine power.

Where does that divine power come from? You know that one of the things that women do very easily—usually far more easily than men—is love. We have the capacity to open our hearts and really love with everything inside of us. Sometimes we might look at this as a weakness. When we give ourselves over to others too easily, we can get hurt. However, regardless of outcomes, regardless of how others may react, I believe that our divine power is all about love. When we love with the power of the divine, nothing can really hurt us. Nothing can touch us. Our love is a gift that we give to the world and to ourselves. When we love fully but wisely, without selfishness and with only pure joy, our love becomes a powerful tool to change our world and the world around us.

When you get right down to it, I don't think there's anything that makes us more powerful in the world than love. All of the money, all of the success—it's all good, and we want it and it's perfectly okay to work toward that. That's the icing on the cake. But the cake—the thing that really matters—is love. It all starts with love.

It doesn't have to be romantic love, although that kind of love can be transformative. It's just about loving: loving mankind, loving the planet, and most of all, loving yourself. It's about living from your heart and approaching everything and everyone from a place of love as often as you can.

Imagine if the entire world operated from a base of this kind of power. There would be no war. Starving children would be fed. We'd all take care of the planet and each other. Suffering wouldn't vanish completely, but much of the pain in the world would if everyone just reached out to help everyone else with love.

You can't change the world—at least not alone—but you can start by changing *your* world. You have the power to shine your love on everyone you know, and everyone you encounter. People will gravitate toward you, because all that love will radiate from you and make everyone you touch, everyone around you, feel good. That good feeling comes directly from your divine power. How amazing, to have the power to brighten people's worlds, to touch their hearts, and to affect their lives.

You do have that power. It's deep inside you, right now, and it wants to come out and shine. I encourage you to embrace that power right now, to know it exists and to claim it. All you need to do is reach inside and look into your heart, and you will find that power within you. Find that light and let it shine out in the world from your heart center. Everybody will feel the vibration, the light, and the love. Nothing is more powerful than that. Nothing transcends darkness and fear more than that light and that love.

And nothing is more beautiful.

WHAT REALLY WORKS FOR ME

Nothing has helped me feel, know, and understand my power more than putting that power to use. My daughter has inspired me to use my power to love, beginning with self-love. You've probably heard the expression "You can't love anyone if you don't love yourself." I want to love my daughter totally and completely, so I focus my power on loving myself, flaws and all.

Because of this, my power to love has grown so much. Not only am I able to love my daughter more deeply and unconditionally but that same power of love has guided me through everything I do, from my work to my relationships. It's almost hard to believe how empowering coming from a place of love can be!

Remember, you are worthy of unconditional love for yourself and from others as well.

Being in a state of love is truly a magical experience. ...

Try it. I know you will *love* it!

Day 24:
I FOLLOW THE HERD.
I LEAD BY EXAMPLE.

You must be the change you wish to see in the world.
— Mahatma Ghandi

As we head into Day 24, I want to congratulate you for how far you have come on our New 10 journey. Think of everything you have accomplished so far over the past few weeks. You've learned to see yourself in a new way, to value yourself and your body, and, most important, to get in touch with your spirit and your soul.

I believe in my heart that this has been working for you and transforming you, that every day, you are becoming more secure in yourself, more powerful—and yes, more beautiful. You are becoming so much more than you ever were in the past. Now you're ready to give something back to the world and the people around you. You're ready to stand up and lead by example.

Why should you put yourself out there in this way? We've all been given certain gifts as women. Now that you're uncovering those gifts that make you special, that make you important and valuable, you're discovering more power than you ever knew you had. But as the saying goes, with great power comes great responsibility. You now have the power to share your gifts with the world to help make it a better place. And you have the power to behave in a way that's worthy of the New 10 you are becoming.

As you get more in touch with your higher self, you develop the strength to hold yourself to a higher standard. When we feel bad about ourselves, many of us engage in negative behaviors to—for lack of a better way of putting it—boost ourselves up and make ourselves feel better, often at others' expense. Maybe we gossip about other people to deflect attention from what we perceive as our own shortcomings. Maybe we treat other people badly to hide our insecurity. Or maybe we just feel too insignificant to say much of anything to try to make a difference.

The good news is, there is no need for this kind of negativity in your life now. Instead, you can become a beacon to others, encouraging them and helping them be their best selves, just as you are becoming your best self.

It's really important that we take this challenge and embrace and accept our power and lead by example. We can lead our children. We can lead our families. We can even lead our friends, our coworkers, even strangers. Because honestly, what we do with our lives and how we live our lives is the best indicator of our inner power and our inner beauty. If we live within our truth—whatever it may be—and radiate that truth, our beauty will shine on everyone we touch.

Being true to ourselves and living with integrity really does make a difference in how others perceive us, not to mention how we perceive ourselves. After all, when we do the right thing, when we feel proud of our actions, we feel good about ourselves. Our self-esteem grows. We stand a little taller, hold our head a little higher, and glow with the knowledge that we are living a good and true life. Because living in our truth brings us back into alignment with our core being, our soul, and our light, living in integrity with our truth really allows us to shine. And when we shine, others see it and experience it and even learn from it, if we let them.

This is where leading by example comes in. Don't be afraid to let your new power, your new strength, shine through. I'm not talking about suddenly "knowing everything" and feeling compelled to share it with everyone. I'm talking about the quiet strength that comes from living a true and honest life and just being there for people, being who you are and being confident in that.

I really encourage you to celebrate the New 10 you are becoming by sharing your gifts with the world and leading by example. Commit yourself to living a little more consciously, with respect for the person you are becoming and the power that she has. You'll notice magical things in your life when you do.

WHAT REALLY WORKS FOR ME

Nothing gave me a better opportunity to lead by example than one of the ugliest, nastiest experiences of my life: my last divorce. I'm sure many of you who have been divorced can relate to this one! Instead of letting my anger swallow me, instead of giving in to my baser instincts, I rose above it. I was challenged to stay true to my integrity, my purpose, and my commitment to helping other women. And I was able to meet that challenge.

Today, I view this painful time as a gift. It helped me become stronger and more beautiful. It challenged me to step up and be the best person I could be. And when I saw what was possible, I became more determined than ever to lead women into their greatest expression of beauty.

It does take courage to lead by example and a willingness to be totally transparent. But the results—the respect you will have for yourself and from others—is totally worth it; nothing will build your sense of self more than being true to your highest self. That's who your soul wants you to be.

And yes, you're worth it!

Day 25:
I HAVE NOTHING TO BE GRATEFUL FOR.
I HAVE EVERYTHING TO BE GRATEFUL FOR.

A pessimist sees only the dark side of the clouds, and mopes; a philosopher sees both sides, and shrugs; an optimist doesn't see the clouds at all—he's walking on them.
— Leonard Louis Levinson

How grateful are you? Do you live in a state of gratitude? Do you recognize what you are blessed with?

These questions are so, so important when it comes to getting in touch with your beautiful spirit. Being grateful has amazing power to transform you and your life. It is such a humbling emotion, but at the same time, it gives you enormous power. We're going to dedicate today to recognizing your blessings and feeling grateful for them.

Maybe you are going through a difficult time and having trouble seeing the blessings in your life. Maybe you don't feel you have very much to be grateful for. Trust me, you do—we all do. You just have to open your eyes, your mind, and your heart to see them.

Sometimes, recognizing a blessing is a matter of perspective. It's a matter of taking yourself out of a situation and asking, "What is the gift in this? What is the blessing in this?" For example, you might not immediately see anything positive in losing a job. But when you step outside the panic and anger and hurt and really look at the situation, you might see it differently. Maybe losing your job will give you an opportunity to find a job that you enjoy more, or to escape a situation that isn't really working for you.

When you can look at a problem that way, when you can see the other side of a situation, you can begin to understand that you are not a victim, that things happen for a reason. And you can be grateful that the universe steps in and takes care of you, even when you don't know exactly why or how.

Of course, gratitude isn't just about finding a new perspective on things that go wrong. It's also about looking at everything that is right in your life—all its blessings—and acknowledging them and giving thanks for them. This is an incredibly powerful thing to do, because when you're experiencing gratitude, when you're thinking about your blessings, it's almost impossible to feel angry, or resentful, or hurt, or afraid, or worried.

Think about what you are grateful for, and you can't help but feel *good.* And when you feel good, you feel beautiful, and you radiate those good feelings and that beauty on everyone around you.

I encourage you to really look at and think about all that is good and beautiful in your life right now. I guarantee you that the more you do this, the more your heart will open, which will bring even more blessings to be grateful for.

Because it is such a powerful force, I want you to make gratitude a part of your daily life. I promise this is not difficult to do, especially if you make it a habit. One thing that I've found works for me is to make a list before I go to bed—either in my head or on a piece of paper—of ten things that I am sincerely, honestly grateful for, and to thank the universe for them.

If you're not sure where to begin to find these things, you can start by thinking about yourself. You're alive, which is an enormous gift and a blessing. You have your breath; you have your mind and your heart. Even if you've been going through a difficult time, you can be grateful that you are strong enough to survive, and smart enough to learn lessons from the experience. You can even be grateful for physical features like beautiful eyes or a good figure, or personality traits like intelligence, compassion, or curiosity.

The point I'm trying to make is that whoever you are and whatever point you're at in your life, you definitely have more than ten things to be grateful for. And the amazing thing is, we haven't even moved beyond yourself to the world around you. When you look past yourself, there are probably more blessings than you can count.

There are the people in your life who matter to you. The beautiful world around you. Even your material possessions. The music you love, the movies and TV shows that entertain you. The water you drink, the air you breathe, the food you eat. You can be grateful for the money that you have, even if it isn't very much. It's still your money, and you still have it.

Most of all, you can be grateful for any experience that has helped you learn and grow, because growing stronger and more beautiful every day is what this journey is all about.

WHAT REALLY WORKS FOR ME

What works for me is to always, always, always remember how lucky I am. By always remembering, I live in a constant state of gratitude.

I have walked through many fires in my life and been transformed by all of them, by the grace of God. So when I think about the hard times, I can't help but see how they helped me to grow and to change into the woman I am today. Even my pain leads me to gratitude. When I experience something difficult, I remember how those hard times transformed me, and I am grateful again that the universe is constantly shaping and molding me into a better, stronger, more beautiful person.

I am grateful for all that I am, for all that I am becoming, and for all that I have ... in the areas of health, wealth, love, family, friends, spirituality, and materially, all of the time.

The more you are sincerely grateful for something, the more of that same something will be attracted to you.

What are you grateful for?

Day 26:
I IGNORE MY HEART.
I LISTEN TO MY HEART.

The intuitive mind is a sacred gift and the rational mind is a faithful servant. We have created a society that honors the servant and has forgotten the gift.
— Albert Einstein

Welcome to a Day 26 in our New 10 journey together. Today is a day we're going to dedicate to a subject you might not normally associate with the overall concept of beauty, or what you think it means to be beautiful. However, it's a special part of each and every one of us that you may be overlooking, despite how enormously important it is. And it deserves to be explored, developed, and celebrated. I'm talking about your intuition.

Since I'm a psychic intuitive, it probably comes as no surprise that I believe strongly in the power of intuition. However, I also believe that, although I am grateful for the intuitive gifts that God has given me, I am not particularly special in this regard. We all have intuition. What makes the difference is recognizing it, as well as knowing and understanding how to use it.

I personally believe that at every moment of every day, we are divinely guided by our own intuitive capacities. The answers and guidance we need to make the right choices in our lives are all there for the taking. The problem, for most of us, is that we have no idea how to access this information, or how to recognize an intuitive message if we happen to receive one. In fact, many women are bombarded by these messages all day long, but have no idea that they have any real meaning or power.

You've probably heard the term *women's intuition* before. Well, there is a good reason for that. As women, we are basically guided by our hearts. And our hearts are really the first place our intuition comes from. Oftentimes, when we get a "hunch" or a "feeling" about something, it is actually our heart sending us a message. The reason we should take these messages seriously is that our hearts do not lie; they can't. Our hearts know right from wrong, they know good from bad, they know truth from falsehood. Yes, they can make mistakes, but only pure and honest ones. So if you feel something in your heart, chances are fairly strong that it is true.

You've no doubt also heard the expression "Listen to your heart." That is the first and easiest way to begin using your intuition. Our hearts are where our souls speak to us and where God speaks to us. If you're looking for guidance or an answer, take a quiet moment and ask your heart to guide you. If you do what your heart tells you to do, you will be following your intuition.

There are actually ways to build this intuitive muscle and train yourself to use and trust your intuition. One thing I have found especially helpful is intuitive journaling. I would really like you to try it.

Get a special journal and, for the next thirty days, complete this exercise every day. Each day I want you to go to a quiet, private spot and ask yourself a question. Then put your hand over your heart, take a deep breath, and allow the answer to come to you through your heart. Write that answer in the journal exactly as it is given to you. Do not censor anything. Do this for thirty days.

At the end of the thirty days go back and read through the journal. There, you will see in black and white (or whatever color you like to write in) the results of your intuition at work. You will discover how many times your intuition was right and see for yourself just how powerful your intuition is.

Once you know that you have this power inside you, you will become more confident as an intuitive being. You will be more willing to listen to that small voice inside you and let it guide you.

The truth is, when we listen to that voice, even if it seems like we're not doing the right thing, there is a reason we are being guided in that particular direction. That's what you need to trust. You need to trust that when you listen to your heart—your intuition—you are always being guided down the right path. Our intuition will tell us when to slow down, or switch gears, or change direction. We always know in our hearts what the right thing to do is, as long as we listen to our internal guidance on a daily basis.

This is an incredibly magical way to live your life, and it's really where the beauty part comes in. You stop chasing after things that won't work or don't matter. You stop seeking counsel from others. You stop looking for outside influences in your life and start looking inward, toward your heart and soul. As you become more confident in yourself and in your ability to guide yourself and make decisions that are good for you, you become empowered and your soul awakens.

And your true beauty shines through.

WHAT REALLY WORKS FOR ME

As a professional intuitive, I've made a career out of listening to my heart. So in this case, this really is "expert advice." Whenever I receive intuitive guidance, it helps me to remember that that guidance is based solely on the present moment. I do not need, nor do I ask for, guidance for future events. I ask to see only the next step to take ... not the whole staircase.

For me, a huge part of intuition is learning to trust in the order of things. And okay, in this case even I am not an expert. I am still striving to trust in the divine timing of things—but more often than not, my intuition tells me to calm down, sit back, and remember that the universe will take care of it.

As I said before, just because I am a professional doesn't mean I have powers that you do not. It's all just a matter of listening to and acting on your intuition. Try it. It is truly empowering!

Day 27:
I HAVE NO IMAGINATION.
I USE MY IMAGINATION.

The best dreams happen when you are awake.
— Cherie Gilderbloom

Welcome to Day 27 of our journey together. I hope you've enjoyed spending the past few days really working on and getting in touch with your spirit. Even though your spirit may not have a physical presence—besides your actual body, of course—I believe a beautiful spirit is probably the most essential aspect of being a New 10. No matter what shape or form your physical body takes, it can't help but be beautiful if your beautiful spirit shines through.

One aspect of a beautiful spirit you might not have thought about is imagination. That isn't a surprise. When we were children, most of our imaginations were probably in overdrive. We pictured ourselves as doctors or movie stars or princesses. We imagined what kind of houses we would live in when we grew up, what kind of places we would visit, the cars we would drive, even what our children would look like. We played games called "let's pretend" and "dress up" and "make-believe" that were completely and totally centered on our imaginations.

But as we grew up and entered the real world, many of us left our imaginations behind. Today, when we drift off like we did as children, we tell ourselves to "snap out of it" and "stop daydreaming." We think of using our imaginations as unproductive, or a waste of time, and an activity that should be avoided.

We don't think of using our imaginations as proper "adult behavior."

Even if we have nothing against the idea of imagination, many more of us simply don't think about it as a viable part of ourselves. In the midst of the day-to-day running of our lives, the practical matters, the dealing with husbands or boyfriends and children and work and errands, who has time to really sit down and imagine? We might catch ourselves doing it accidentally from time to time, but we probably would never do it deliberately.

I'm here to tell you that you absolutely should. When you imagine something, when you drift off into a daydream, you aren't just wasting time. That daydream is actually your soul trying to tell you something. It may be trying to tell you what it thinks is beautiful, or what it wants more deeply than anything else, or where it wants you to pay some special attention.

If you're like most adult women, you may be missing these messages. You may not value your imagination, let alone use it. But if you're shutting off that part of yourself—of your spirit—you're actually blocking something that's important, valuable, and beautiful.

I want you to take this day to get in touch with what your soul is trying to tell you through your imagination. Take some time, even if it's only a few minutes, to let your mind wander. Let your soul take you places where you've never been before. Try to honor and remember what you see, what you feel, what you hear, and what you sense. Remember not to censor what your imagination is telling you or where it takes you. Remember that your imagination is actually your soul talking, trying to guide you to a higher expression in life.

Also remember that if you can see it and imagine it, you can make it true. It's important to dream, and to dream big, so that we know and understand what our souls really want for us. You may have heard about the power of visualization, and we'll be talking more about it later in the book. Well, visualization is just a targeted way of daydreaming ... or imagining. Sometimes to reach our fullest potential, we need to be able to see what it will be. We need to use our imaginations to make that happen.

Imagining isn't something just children do. It's also a really big part of becoming a totally empowered and awakened woman. Feel free to imagine who and what you want to be, what you want from life, whatever your mind wants to imagine, wherever you are right now. Take some time every week to let your mind roam freely, wherever it wants to go. You will start to learn things about yourself that you never knew before.

And if you honor what you learn, you will grow more beautiful.

WHAT REALLY WORKS FOR ME

I have learned to take my imagination very seriously.

Why? Well, when I allow myself to daydream or imagine, I learn what my heart desires, I see what I am capable of becoming, and I remember that nothing is too good for me to desire or achieve. In other words, my imagination connects me to my soul. Often what I imagine is what my soul is asking for. Imagination is the way I get the message when I am otherwise too busy to notice.

Because of this, I make time to use my imagination. When my normal, everyday mind feels limited—which can happen—I curl up in a favorite chair and just let my mind wander. When I use my imagination and put my heart into it, I can see possibilities that are unlimited, yet very achievable.

Just imagine the possibilities if you did this too. ...

Day 28:
I DON'T WANT MUCH. I WANT IT ALL!

Life has no limitations, except the ones you make.
— Leo Brown

As we continue our exploration of our beautiful spirits, I have a question for you. Do you know what your spirit really, truly wants for you? And are you honoring that in the way you live your life and approach each day?

Chances are, you may not be. Because whatever you are doing right now, your spirit wants you to ask for more.

This seems to be an especially difficult area for a lot of women. Maybe as a child you learned not to ask for more—that it wasn't polite, or ladylike, or nice. Maybe you wanted a toy, or a second helping, or to stay up later, and were told no. Maybe it happened more than once. You learned it was best to be happy with what you had, to settle for less, to accept things as they were.

Today I'm going to tell you to do the opposite. I want you to ask for more from the universe. The only catch is, I also want you to ask for more from yourself.

Our spirits really want us to live our best lives possible. They don't want us to settle for less; they want us to reach for the stars and experience as many wonderful, beautiful, amazing things as we possibly can. However, we're not really able to live at that level unless we are constantly willing to expand our thoughts, expand our emotions, expand our belief systems, and expand our paradigms to be more all-encompassing. We have to start thinking in bigger ways and expecting more from ourselves. When we do, we get more from the universe as well.

The universe is a place of abundance. Everything you could possibly want or need is there for the taking. But some of us just don't feel right about the taking part. We feel that taking for ourselves means taking *away* from someone else—that our abundance is someone else's scarcity. Luckily, this isn't true.

The universe is unlimited—it's infinite—so we aren't taking anything away from anybody else by wanting things for ourselves. We aren't being greedy. The more you create for yourself, the more you serve as an example to others of what is possible for them (remember that from a few chapters back?), and the more you pave the way for others to create more for themselves too. That's called a win-win situation.

How do we gain access to all that the universe is offering us? We need to really start expanding our mind-sets, to expect more, to ask for more, and most of all to be willing to receive more and give more. Because the more we give, the more we receive.

It's really about having an attitude of openness—about saying yes where you might otherwise say no. Every time you say yes, you open the door to new experiences that will enrich you and help you grow. Instead of being closed off from the universe, saying yes opens you up to the universe and all it has to offer you. That's not to say that everything you try, that every new experience, will be right for you. But as long as you listen to your intuition and remember to stay true to yourself and your core values and beliefs, every single experience you have will expand your universe that much more.

There is no reason not to open yourself up to all that's available to you in this lifetime. If you want to live your best life, you need to take advantage of everything that is here for you right now. I really encourage you to expand your thinking. You deserve to have it all, be it all, and do it all. All you need to do is be open to it all and let yourself experience it all, and I promise you will benefit from it all.

As you expand your heart, your mind, and your world, your spirit becomes that much more fulfilled. It shines through and lights up your entire being, not to mention it shines your light on everyone around you.

This is where real beauty comes from. It comes from embracing the universe with open arms, loving life, loving yourself, and loving everyone you see. As women, we have an amazing capacity to love and to operate from a place of love. If you approach new things and situations with love, your true beauty can only grow.

WHAT REALLY WORKS FOR ME

I started to view my life and my potential as being without limits. Every time a limiting thought popped into my head, I reminded myself to value what my heart guides me to do, be, and have. It didn't happen automatically; it took years for me to "re-learn" my desire to have it all when I was still a child. But over time, with practice, I learned that wanting to have it all is a good and positive thing. Today, I allow myself to want to have it all, and to pursue that desire.

I don't always get what I want the minute I think of it. The universe doesn't work that way! But I don't forget. I keep my cherished dreams close to my heart until they come true.

Another thing that works for me is trying to stay away from negativity as much as I can. I am careful to avoid the news and newspapers and those negative headlines on the Internet.

The heart does not lie. ... If you allow it to think for you in terms of your "brilliance," you will also find yourself acting from the heart, from a place of greater love, joy, and peace. This helps to speed up the manifestation process, because you eliminate the negative energy that can get in the way. So whatever *you* want, whatever *you* really desire, remember, it can be yours.

Because you deserve to have it all too!

Day 29:
I CHEAT MYSELF.
I TREAT MYSELF.

Hello and welcome to Day 29. You know, we've been together on this journey for almost a month now. I'm wondering how much you've changed since that first day when we set out on this adventure together. Are you feeling more empowered, more awakened, and most of all, more divinely beautiful? Have you learned to appreciate and celebrate the amazing, incredible, beautiful woman that you are? I know in my heart that you have, or at least that you are getting there. Today we're going to talk about how to show that beautiful woman some appreciation—and to let her spirit soar. We're going to talk about the gift of giving to ourselves romantically.

Maybe you have a romantic partner in your life; maybe you are single. It really doesn't matter. This isn't about depending on someone else to fill our lives with joy and romance. This is about using our own power and our own self-knowledge—a depth of knowledge no one else can possibly have about what brings us joy—to romance ourselves first.

Ask yourself, Do you honor your romantic nature? Do you light candles for yourself? Do you put on romantic music just for you? Do you fill your house with your favorite flowers? I do. I love flowers, I think they're beautiful, and I love what they add to my home. I don't have an issue with buying them for myself. Yes, you might have someone in your life who you hope will buy flowers for you. But waiting for someone else to give you what you want is not what your spirit wants from you—or for you.

Of course, if you have a romantic partner in your life, buying your own flowers or lighting your own candles will give that partner an opportunity to see what makes you happy, what you love, what makes your spirit soar. And if he (or she) is sensitive to your needs, he (or she) will make a mental note of what makes you happy and use that information in the future.

However, that is not what this day is about. This day is not about teaching others to do things for you. This is about teaching *you* to do things for you. This is about realizing that your spirit really deserves what it wants, and that it is your responsibility to create and give yourself what you deserve. Being romanced by another person is obviously one of the great joys of life. But romancing ourselves, our spirits, and our souls is even more important. It is about valuing yourself. About respecting yourself. And, more than anything, about loving yourself.

Today I want you to set aside some time to romance yourself and celebrate the beautiful woman you are becoming every day. It doesn't have to be about spending a lot of money. If you can't afford to buy flowers, pick some wildflowers at a local park, or just buy an inexpensive bouquet at the grocery store. When you get home, put on some soft music that makes you happy. Turn down the lights and light some candles. If you have children or other people around who might not understand why the whole house is dark, sneak off to the bathroom and soak in a bubble bath surrounded by candles. You can even play music in there, and if you're feeling really, really decadent, treat yourself to a glass of wine or champagne.

Or maybe, if you're more of an outdoorsy, active type of person, take yourself for a walk in nature, through the woods or along the beach. Bring your favorite quiet music, or just listen to the sounds of nature and your own thoughts. Give that gift to yourself of time alone, doing something you love that makes you feel good.

I promise you, you'll notice a joy in your spirit and a feeling of well-being within yourself when you give yourself this gift. What it's really about is the gift of time—time to focus on you and no one but you. Time to take care of yourself as opposed to taking care of others. Time to pamper yourself and, yes, to love yourself.

Chances are, you will feel so good after romancing yourself that you will want to do it again. So make a date with yourself once a week to just focus on you. Your spirit will thank you, and your beauty will grow.

The true, inner and outer beauty of a New 10.

WHAT REALLY WORKS FOR ME

It's actually really simple. I pay attention to my life. I try to be conscious at all times. And although I don't like to dwell on the negative, I try to be honest with myself: if something is missing, if I need something I am not getting, I will be open to that realization.

To do that, I had to let go of all the guilt that I (and most women) have around the idea of having needs that are valid and real. But in exploring my heart and soul so deeply, I learned that it is completely normal and healthy to have needs—and very *un*healthy to deny myself the things I need.

Once I determine that something is missing from my life, I open my mind and my soul to ways that I can give them to myself instead of waiting to receive them from others and feeling angry or disappointed when I don't.

This really helps me feel in control of creating my own beautiful life. I take full responsibility for my own happiness and experience more of it as a result ... and you can too!

Day 30:
LIFE IS A TRAGEDY.
LIFE IS A COMEDY.

Celebrate your success and find humor in your failures. Don't take yourself so seriously. Loosen up and everyone around you will loosen up. Have fun and always show enthusiasm. When all else fails, put on a costume and sing a silly song.
— Sam Walton (founder of Wal-Mart)

Over the past few weeks, we've talked about a lot of serious subjects. We've dealt with our souls and our spirits, our minds and our bodies, and how we can find the beauty in all of them. Today, as we close out our focus on the spirit, I'd like to lighten the mood a little and talk about an aspect of our spirit that is just as important as all that serious stuff like self-love and living by example. I want to talk about your sense of humor.

How often do you laugh? Some people are lucky enough to laugh loudly, laugh hard, and laugh often—even several times a day. But others are so overwhelmed by their problems and the stresses of life that they hardly laugh at all. If that sounds like you, it is time to lighten up. Not only is laughter fun and a great tension breaker but it also opens us up, changes our perspective, and allows good things and change to happen.

The world is full of things to laugh at if you only look at them from the right perspective. Some people have a real gift for this. They tend to be the people who love comedy, who love to tell and hear jokes, who will always pick a funny movie over a drama, and who always seem to be laughing, even when things aren't going particularly well for them. If you are one of those people, know that your sense of humor is a gift and part of what makes you beautiful. Your ability to find joy and fun even in life's darkest moments will help not only you but everyone around you.

If your sense of humor is not in top form, don't worry about it. You can develop it. Practice looking for the funny side of things. Rent some funny movies that you like and watch them again, paying special attention to where and how they make you laugh. Spend time with people who are lighthearted and funny—the experience will rub off on you. They can help you change your perspective, because humor is all about perspective. It's about seeing the lighter side of a situation, no matter what it is.

Even our own problems and challenges can be viewed with a sense of humor, as impossible as that may sound. Try imagining yourself as a character in a sitcom or movie, having the exact same problems and challenges that you do right now. Now think about how those problems would play out for your "character." Not only will you be able to see the humor in your situation but you might also be able to see some solutions you hadn't thought of. After all, comedies usually have happy endings. Seeing the entertainment value in your own situation can help point the way to your own happy ending.

Our spirits want us to live our lives in joy. We actually have joy guides all around us, but when we're feeling down or miserable or overwhelmed, we just don't know they are there or how to find them. When times get tough, instead of dwelling on how horrible things are, I'd like you to call on your joy guides and ask them to help you see the lighter side. If you absolutely cannot see the lighter side of your own situation, then ask them to help you remember a joke or a funny moment that is going to help you smile and laugh. The idea is to change your aura and your energy around whatever is bothering you and truly lighten up.

Life can be challenging, but it doesn't have to be as difficult as it seems. We have the power within us to take responsibility for how we respond to our challenges and lessons. We don't have to be miserable. We can learn to look at our problems from a higher, lighter, more joyful and humorous perspective.

It will help those problems diminish—while our beauty only grows.

WHAT REALLY HELPS ME

I admit it: I struggle with this one. Sometimes I am just way too serious!

I am so lucky I have my daughter. She helps me see myself through someone else's eyes—and trust me, there are times when *she* thinks I am downright hilarious, even if I can't quite see what is so funny. But seriously, my daughter has taught me to laugh at myself when things get hard, which things have a tendency to do. I think I have grown a lot in this area over her twelve years of guidance, because she comments a lot on how much lighter and happier I am.

Of course, my twelve-year-old child is not responsible for bringing laughter into my life—I am. When the going gets really tough, I turn to the things I know will make me laugh. I love comedies, and they help me get over myself when I need to. I keep DVDs of TV shows and movies that I know will make me laugh on hand for those times when I need them.

Another thing I do is challenge myself to go through life's next lesson just a little more gracefully. This may require some humor, but I am worth it ... and so are you!

MY LIFE IS ORDINARY.
MY LIFE IS EXTRAORDINARY.

> *Start living now. Stop saving the good china for a special occasion. Stop withholding your love until the special person materializes. Every day you are alive is a special occasion. Every minute, every breath, is a gift from God.*
> — Mary Manin Morrissey

By this point in the book, you've no doubt learned that our beauty isn't manifested just in our faces and bodies. You know that your mind and spirit are also essential to your beauty, especially to becoming the New 10 that you are inside. Now, as we move into the last part of our journey together, I want you to take that beauty you're feeling and radiating inside and out and use it. I want you to live a boldly beautiful life.

What exactly does that mean? It means approaching every day and every situation from a place of strength, openness, and grace. It means having the confidence to live the life that you want and go after the things that make you happy. It means knowing that you deserve the best and living as if it is your right. Because you know what? It is your right.

Of course, like everything else in this book, living a boldly beautiful life takes practice.

It may feel strange to carry the sense that you are entitled to the best in everything that you do.

It may not feel natural to expect good things to happen to you.

But they will if you let them. It's time to learn together how to let them happen.

Over our final ten days together, we will focus on how you can live a boldly beautiful life. How you can attract the things you so richly deserve. And how you can radiate your true beauty wherever you go, whatever you do.

You are a New 10, and a boldly beautiful life is the life you are meant to have.

So keep reading … and start living.

Day 31:
I AM UNCONSCIOUS.
I AM CONSCIOUS.

Light tomorrow with today.
— Elizabeth Barrett Browning

I want to begin this last part of our journey by talking about what I believe could be the most important aspect of living the life you deserve. I want to talk about living consciously.

Becoming more conscious is an essential part of living a life that is divinely guided—and, of course, beautiful.

I understand that you may not really know what it means to "live consciously," or to "become more conscious," so I will take some time to explain it here.

Being conscious means being awake and aware. That is something you probably think you are all the time, except, of course, when you're sleeping.

The problem for many of us is that that isn't exactly true. You might be surprised to learn that a lot of our behavior is actually automatic. More often than not, we respond and act without thinking, because actively thinking all the time takes energy and effort.

Have you ever been driving somewhere you've been hundreds of times before and missed your exit? Or set out to do something and suddenly wondered, "What exactly am I doing?" Those are both examples of living "on autopilot," without thinking. Sometimes we rely so heavily on our routines, and on previous experiences, that we have very little awareness of what is going on in a particular moment.

When this happens, we miss a lot. We fail to experience the beauty of the moment. We fail to be engaged in the moment. How can we possibly get the most out of a moment that we are not engaged in? Trust me: it's difficult to get the most out of something when you don't even know you're there!

But there are other, even more destructive ways we respond automatically, without thinking.

Sometimes we have automatic responses to bad news or negative experiences. Maybe you always lash out in anger, or retreat into yourself. Maybe whenever something goes wrong, you automatically blame yourself and start beating up on yourself. These are automatic responses too, and examples of living *un*consciously.

When we become more conscious, we can stop these processes in their tracks. Becoming more conscious means becoming more aware of who we are, what we're doing, and why we're doing it. It's not about becoming aware of just our actions, but of the reasons behind those actions. It's about asking yourself why you behaved in a certain way, or reacted in a certain way. And it's about waiting for the divine guidance you need to get the most out of every moment—even a negative one. Because there is beauty in every moment of your life.

The first step in becoming more conscious is simply to question what you do. When you ask questions, you can't help becoming more aware of the thought processes and patterns that have ruled your life. The more you're willing to learn, and the more you're willing to open yourself up to, the more aware you will become. And a space will open up to let that guidance in.

Right now, I want you to set the intention to become more conscious and to become more aware and do whatever you can to help yourself grow and evolve in that way. It may sound like a difficult proposition—after all, learning to break old patterns and be conscious in every moment isn't going to happen automatically. But if you remind yourself each day that this is the goal you are aiming for, if you remind yourself as you go through the day to be present in each moment and really think about what you are experiencing, I promise you will notice a change.

You will live with more grace and more beauty.

There is also an important tool that can do a lot to help you accomplish this goal. I've found meditation to be a good way to become more conscious as a woman and as an individual. Just taking those few minutes every day to quiet my thoughts has helped me center myself, become more aware of myself, and let divine guidance come to me. With all the other benefits of meditation we've already talked about, I can't stress enough how much this simple act can add to your daily life.

We have come so far together; I promise you it is within your power to take this very important step. I want to applaud you for all your efforts so far, and to remind you that I'm with you on this journey. I'm constantly learning to become more conscious myself. This is not something I'm preaching and teaching, this is a process I'm sharing with you. It amazes me daily and weekly what I learn about myself—but the best part is, I'm able to make adjustments accordingly. It's amazing how these little changes benefit me and everyone around me.

I guarantee the same will happen for you. And it will be beautiful.

WHAT REALLY WORKS FOR ME

As I mentioned before, I have found meditation to be a really powerful tool in this arena. Just that act of making the time, of *consciously* quieting those voices around me, allows me to separate what is real from what is not and what matters from what is trivial, and to bring myself back in line with reality. Since I meditate every day, I am able to stay conscious almost all the time, save a few especially trying periods when I just get too busy and overwhelmed.

I find guided meditations helpful in focusing my energy where it needs to be and getting me past blockages and rough patches. By simply following their lead, I am taken on a journey that I know will get me where I need to go. I really like the "Seeds of Enlightenment" meditation CDs; they are extremely helpful when it comes to both surrendering and awakening. You can order them at www.learningstrategies.com. I hope you enjoy them as much as I have and still do.

Day 32:
I AM A DOER.
I AM A BE-ER.

The snow goose need not bathe to make itself white.
Neither need you do anything but be yourself.
— Lao-Tse

Hello and welcome to Day 32 of our journey together. As we continue to learn to live lives filled with beauty, I want to ask you an important question. How much of your time do you spend not doing, but simply being?

As women, we spend much of our time doing. If we're mothers, we spend time taking care of our families: shopping for them, feeding them, keeping their clothes clean and their bodies healthy, and getting them to all the places they need to go. If we're married or in relationships, we take care of our partners. We worry about their emotional needs; we take care of and do things for them.

Even if we're single and childless, that doesn't mean we do any less. We do things for our bosses, our coworkers, or our clients. We do things for our friends and maybe our families. We do our jobs. And of course, we still need to do things for ourselves. We take care of the day-to-day chores we need to survive, from paying the bills to taking care of our cars. We need to keep a roof over our head and food on our table.

In other words, we have a lot to do.

Which doesn't leave a whole lot of time to simply be.

What does it mean to just be? For starters, it means taking some time for yourself when you don't have to *do* anything. It means taking a quiet moment by yourself, just being alone with your own thoughts. It means looking out the window at the clouds rolling by, or the rain falling, or the wind rustling through the trees. It means curling up with a good book or a magazine. It means sitting and listening to music. It means walking down the beach, or through the woods, or even through the streets of your town—not with any particular destination or purpose in mind, but just to enjoy the fresh air.

In other words, it means doing whatever "doing nothing" means to you.

Of course, you might read this and think that by "being," I'm actually talking about being lazy.

After all, "doing" means having a purpose. It means being productive. So would "being" be the exact opposite?

I want to assure you that nothing could be further from the truth.

When we take time to just be, we take care of ourselves. We nurture our spirits and our souls by giving them a chance to rest. We give ourselves the time we need to regroup and revitalize, to reconnect with ourselves. When we take time to be, we take time to step outside the craziness of our lives.

Taking time to just be gives our bodies and our souls the break we need to improve our focus, our concentration, and our mood. That makes the *doing* part of our lives much more joyful and much easier. It's actually essential as women to learn to take this time and give this gift to ourselves, so that we have more to give to our loved ones and our jobs and everything else in our lives.

The most important thing that happens when we learn to just be has nothing to do with how we perform when we do, or how we give to others. It has to do with the gift we give ourselves by getting to know ourselves better.

By taking this time to honor yourself and your spirit and your soul, you give yourself an incredible gift. You start to really understand who you are and feel more comfortable in your own skin. You start to feel more comfortable being alone, because you learn to experience the fulfillment that comes with being able to spend high-quality time with yourself. It helps you grow stronger, more centered, and yes, more beautiful.

This may be a big challenge for you at first, to take fifteen minutes or a half hour out of your busy day and practice just being. But I want you to try it. Whatever sounds appealing to you, whether it's going for a walk or having a cup of tea by the fire, I want you to carve out some time for you. And do it every day. I promise it will get easier; you will get more comfortable and get more out of it every time.

Above all, just remember that you need and deserve this time to live your most beautiful life. And as a New 10, that's the kind of life you should be living.

WHAT REALLY WORKED FOR ME

My home is my sanctuary, but since I do everything there, it's a lot of other things too. It's my office, my gym, and even my meditation space. Sometimes for me to just "be," I need to "be" someplace else! That means taking time for myself and getting out and enjoying the world around me.

Some days that means going out to dinner with my daughter, some days it means being with friends, other days it includes dates with my boyfriend or going shopping ... alone (which I love to do!).

Whether you're happiest curled up in the corner with a book or out on the town, make sure you take time for yourself. It really does replenish my spirit, and I know it will do the same for you. Try it. ... You're worth it.

Day 33:
I LIVE IN THE PAST.
I LIVE IN THE NOW.

We can only Be Here Now when we accept instantly our moment-by-moment emotional experience.
— Gita Bellin

Right now, as we begin Day 33, I want you to stop for a moment. I want you to take a long, deep breath and really feel the oxygen as it fills your lungs. Now I want you to look at the world around you. Look at the sunlight, or the moonlight, or the clouds, or the rain, or the light as it pours in through the window. Right now, wherever you are, I want you to appreciate this moment for all of its beauty, and for all the possibilities it holds. It's your moment. It's happening right now. And you can make it whatever you want it to be.

This is what's called living in the now. And it's an essential part of living a boldly beautiful life.

One of my favorite sayings is "It is a brand new day, so let's embrace it for what it is." It's true—every new day is a gift. Regardless of what happened yesterday, or last week, or last month, or even last year, every new day is an opportunity to start over and to leave the past behind. It's a chance to start completely fresh, to put all you have learned so far about living as a New 10 to work, and to see where this beautiful new day takes you.

Of course, it can be tempting to think about where this beautiful day might take us tomorrow, and the next day, and next week and next month and even next year. And it's perfectly okay to dream about the future. That's positive and healthy and a great way to set goals.

But it's not okay to worry or to dwell about what might happen someday, or to spend all of our time thinking about what is to come instead of what is happening right now. When we get too caught up in the future, it's just as bad as staying mired in our past.

We miss the gift of now.

Now is an incredible gift—filled with promise and possibility.

By living in the present moment with more awareness and more consciousness, we make the most of each moment we are given on this earth. When we're busy making the most of every precious moment we have, the future has a way of taking care of itself.

We have much to learn from the present. If we can keep our awareness in the moment, and keep our consciousness focused on the moment we are in, we are putting ourselves in the right frame of mind to live a boldly beautiful life. Instead of thinking, "I wish I hadn't yelled at my daughter yesterday" or worrying about what's going to happen at work tomorrow, we can fully experience *right now*. What can we do to get the most out of this moment? How can we best appreciate the gift of being here, of being alive, of being present?

If we manage to live in the moment and be conscious in the moment, we will be open to divine guidance. The universe will lead us exactly where we need to go.

Living with this level of awareness and consciousness constantly feeds us enlightenment, information, and inspiration. It's where our most inspired ideas come from. It's also where our joy comes from and where our happiness comes from. When we're just focusing on the moment, there is nothing wrong in our world. We are safe. We are happy. Everything is good and beautiful. The more we are able to focus our energy on living in the now, the more we will feel it internally, and the more our life will reflect it externally.

I encourage you to do everything you can do to remind yourself to live in the now. Don't dwell on the past; you can learn from it and move on. Don't worry about the future; make the right choices in the moment you have and it will take care of itself. If you open yourself up in this way, and permit all the possibilities of life to come to you, you will realize that you are not alone. You are always being guided toward your highest potential. It's up to you to take responsibility for your now moments and live them to the fullest.

They are your gift from God, and they are yours to make beautiful.

WHAT REALLY WORKS FOR ME

This is another instance where meditation has proven to be a lifesaver. Whether my mind is stuck on some past event or racing around thinking about what might happen in the future, that is obviously not where I want to be. But I am human, so of course it happens!

When it does, meditation brings me back into the moment—back into the now. It helps me regain my center and my perspective, as well as being both calming and energizing. By meditating daily, I make sure I never stray too far from the now ... even when I do stray.

You might remember a few days ago I told you about the meditation CDs "Seeds of Enlightenment," which I have found incredibly helpful. They have a specific meditation called "Trust and Surrender" that helps me come back to the present moment whenever I find myself stressing about the future. Again, you can find them at www.learningstrategies.com.

Day 34:
I DON'T WANT TO GROW OLD.
I CAN'T WAIT TO GROW OLD.

I have often wondered how every man loves himself more than all the rest of men, yet sets less value on his own opinion of himself than on the opinion of others.
— Marcus Aurelius

As we begin our final week together, I want to tackle a subject that strikes fear in the hearts of women from all walks of life, especially when they think about beauty.

I'm talking about growing older.

We all know in our minds that none of us should fear growing old, especially when you think about the alternative. But for many of us, just the word *aging* represents the loss of femininity, of sexual power, and of beauty itself—which can be a pretty frightening scenario.

Of course, thanks to the wonders of modern science, many women no longer have to get old at all—at least not in the natural sense that God intended. We can get rid of our wrinkles with Botox injections, suck away the extra pounds that can come with age with liposuction, keep our hair long and thick with extensions, and even have cocktails of "bio-identical hormones" specially whipped up to keep our bodies "forever young."

Of course, all this agelessness costs money. It can be painful. But so many women are spending tens of thousands of dollars to hold off Father Time that in some areas, it's difficult to find a woman over fifty who hasn't had anything "done." In places like this, mothers look "younger" than their own adult daughters, and seeing a forty-five-year-old woman trying to look like a twenty-five-year-old is a common sight.

However, I think it's also a sad sight.

Aging can be beautiful. As we age, we gain wisdom. We gain character. And we gain a deeper, more honest beauty than we had at twenty-five.

Part of that beauty comes from really knowing and accepting ourselves. Part of it comes from the many experiences we've had, including the pain and the heartbreak that have expanded our hearts and our minds and helped us to grow far, far beyond the women we were when we were younger.

Of course, if you are a young woman right now, you have every right to be beautiful too, and to be beautiful right now and enjoy all that your youth has to offer you. Just remember these lessons for when you get older.

The rest of us would probably tell our younger friends that life only gets better as we age. That, regardless of extra pounds or wrinkles or gray hairs, we would never go back. The wisdom we've gained and the experiences we've had are too precious to even think about giving up.

However, it can still be difficult to see those things as beautiful in a culture that seems to prize youth above everything else.

As women, we don't need to buy into that mind-set. We don't need to spend thousands of dollars to try to stop the march of time either. This is not to say you can't indulge in a cosmetic improvement if you want to. If you have the money and think it's worth the investment, there's nothing wrong with spending the money if it makes you feel good.

But the important thing is how you feel inside, not outside. The important thing is that you know and accept in your heart that all the money in the world can't change some things—and one of the things we can't change is that every year, with a little luck, we will all get older.

What we can do, all of us, is change how we feel about aging and how we perceive getting older. If we can embrace our age and the wisdom that it brings us, and allow that wisdom to shine through, then aging can be beautiful. If we allow our spirits to come through and express them boldly, and if we can really feel and revel in the beauty that is within all of us, we actually will appear younger. That kind of beauty doesn't take a plastic surgeon. It just takes the right attitude.

If you really want to age gracefully and age beautifully, don't try to fight what is. Instead, strive to serenely accept what is for the gift that it is.

Remember, just being the best you can be, loving yourself unconditionally, and expressing your spirit gives you more power and beauty than you ever could have had at twenty-five. And when you reach that point where you fully accept and love yourself for who you are, your light will radiate from you like sunshine and you will literally glow with beauty, regardless of your age.

And maybe even because of it.

WHAT REALLY WORKS FOR ME

As I mentioned before, I never really felt truly beautiful until after I turned forty, so maybe I had a bit of a head start in this area. The fact that I spent so many of my younger years beating up on myself and my appearance makes getting older a lot easier. I feel more beautiful as I gain wisdom, as I gain spirituality, as I become a better, stronger person. I can actually feel myself growing more beautiful each day (okay, except on those "bad" days we all have). And that makes getting older a lot easier.

I also take care of myself and work to maintain my looks. I take pride in my appearance and make the most of what God gave me. I forgive myself for not being perfect. But I think what really makes growing older so easy for me is that I have so much to look forward to. I know my greatest accomplishments and happiest days lie ahead, which makes growing older pretty exciting.

That's my key. It can be yours too.

Day 35:
WHEN THINGS GO WRONG, I GO CRAZY! WHEN THINGS GO WRONG, I AM CALM.

> *If you attack apparent negativity, you merely find and inflame the source. It's always better to take the positive in any conflict. If you genuinely love, or at least send kind thoughts to a thing, it will change before your eyes.*
> — John and Lyn St. Clair-Thomas,
> Eyes of the Beholder

Welcome to Day 35 of the New 10 beauty campaign. We've got only five days left together after today, so I really hope these chapters are helping you embrace and celebrate your true beauty in your mind, body, and spirit.

For the past few days, we've been concentrating on living a boldly beautiful life—on carrying that sense of peace, strength, and beauty with us wherever we go. However, there are times when shining that inner beauty on everyone around us is a little more difficult than others. After all, how do we live a boldly beautiful life when we're upset or angry?

Anger can be an ugly emotion. When we're angry, we can say ugly things to people that we regret later. We can lash out and cause pain. If we don't take our anger out on others, we can take it out on ourselves instead. Obviously, this kind of ugliness doesn't really fit in with the idea of a boldly beautiful life. But bad things happen to everyone, even those of us who are empowered and enlightened and in touch with our most beautiful selves.

How do we cope when things really go wrong—when people betray our trust, when we are profoundly hurt or disappointed—in a way that doesn't compromise our New 10 ideals?

It all starts with something that's called nonviolent communication.

As divinely empowered and awakened women, it's really important for us to learn how to communicate in a nonviolent manner. I don't just mean communicating without physical violence; most (but not all!) women are not physically violent, even in the worst of circumstances. I am, however, talking about taking the emotional violence out of our interactions, even when things are difficult and people let us down.

Nonviolent communication means communicating responsively with people who hurt us or make us angry, and striving to do it in a loving manner. It means taking responsibility for our own feelings in our own lives—after all, no one can *really* affect us that negatively if we don't allow them to. It means knowing we are responsible for what we create in our lives, and also for how we treat other people. Being angry or upset is no excuse for being cruel or emotionally violent.

Does this mean that when someone violates our trust or does something nasty to us, we need to keep our mouths shut and simply take it? Not at all. We can express our truth and we can tell people how we feel. That's not the issue. The question is not what we say, but how we say it—and the feelings behind it when we say it.

By this point in our journey, you should feel confident in who you are. You should feel like you have a right to your feelings and like your feelings are not "bad" or even "good"; they are simply there and have a right to be there.

Most of all, you should feel empowered.

The great thing about being empowered is that you don't have to shout to be heard. You don't have to make a scene to command attention. All you need to do is take a few moments—especially when you're emotionally charged—to take a deep breath and calm down before you speak. Think about what you really want to accomplish when you address someone who has wronged or upset you. Think about their position, their feelings, and how you want to be perceived.

Then make your case in the simplest, clearest language possible. You can be completely nonthreatening but also totally clear and completely firm. Remember, you have a right to your opinion. You have a right to make your case. You have a right to be heard, even if you do not "win." There is no reason to lose control.

At its heart, nonviolent communication really is about being more aware and more conscious and thinking before you say something. After we say something to somebody, we can never take it back. And when we let bad feelings provoke us into lashing out, whatever we do to another person has a way of coming back and affecting us tenfold.

Instead, strive to communicate with love and integrity. When we work to inspire other people, to see the best in other people, and to affirm that other people are good and true and also have only the best intentions, we're actually doing the same thing for ourselves.

And we're making all of our worlds a lot more beautiful.

WHAT REALLY WORKED FOR ME

It all came down to one very important decision. I chose to live as a "queen" and give up being a "drama queen," pure and simple. You can be one or the other, but not both.

Let me explain. When things don't go her way, a drama queen lets everyone know about it. She defines herself by what is wrong in her life—to the point where it can seem like she actually enjoys the problems that bring her so much attention.

Often, this type of behavior comes from a place of insecurity. A drama queen isn't sure she deserves to be heard, so she yells to make sure that she is. She doesn't trust that the universe is looking out for her, so when she doesn't get what she wants, she gets angry.

On the other hand, a queen is regal, calm, and in control. This is because, as a queen, she is being taken care of. She knows that things will go wrong from time to time, but that this is all part of life. As a queen, she takes bad news gracefully, and when she has to set boundaries, she is absolutely firm, but never nasty or condescending. She doesn't need to be. She knows she has a divine right to be heard.

I've made my choice. Not that I never have a drama queen moment, but I do my best to live as a queen. So now, the only question is … Whom do you choose to be?

Day 36:
JUST SAY NO.
JUST SAY YES!

*You are a trust fund baby of the Universe. Your only job
is to decide how much you want that trust fund
to be worth; and then be willing to receive it.*
— Sonia Choquette

Wow. It's Day 36, and our time together is starting to draw to a close. I want our final few days of this journey to be about helping you access your divine power to make your life as beautiful as it can possibly be. I want you to be able to open those doors that you might not have even known were closed—or even known were there in the first place—to all the possibilities behind them.

Today, I'm going to introduce you to the most powerful word in the universe.

Ready? Here it is.

It's *YES*.

Of course you probably say yes often. You say it every day, several times a day—to that second cup of coffee, to your children when they ask if you'll help them with their homework, to your partner when he offers a back rub. And in thousands of other situations all day long.

However, you might see a different picture if you think about how often you say no. How often you turn down an opportunity to go somewhere new, try something new, break out of your everyday routine.

It might happen more often than you imagine.

It's not a surprise, really. The word *no* is a safe word. It means staying where you feel in control and safe and comfortable.

But it also means closing a door. And when you do, you stop whatever opportunity was behind that door—an adventure, or growth, or possibility—in its tracks.

When you say no, you're turning your back on something the universe is offering you. Something that, just maybe, might be there to help you grow or change or learn something important about yourself.

In which case the word *no* may be safe ... but may also be a little stifling.

Now, *yes,* on the other hand ... well, *yes* can definitely be scary. Some of us just don't feel comfortable accepting anything, as if any gift is too much. So we say no whenever we are offered something.

For others, it's a matter of being afraid to open the door to whatever is on the other side. Who knows what that might be? It might be dangerous! So we say no.

Of course, to experience something you've never experienced before, to meet a new person, to learn a new skill, to see a new place, to do anything at all, you first have to say yes.

What kind of life you live from this day forward has a lot to do with the word *yes* and learning to say it whenever you can. Ask yourself right now: How willing are you to open up your arms to the universe, to receiving all the things you deserve? You can't do it without saying yes.

Because although the universe will certainly offer these things to you, only you can say yes to them and allow them into your life.

When you say yes to the universe and to all that you need and want and desire, when you say yes to all of your dreams and goals, you enable them to come true. They can't possibly come true if you say no.

So the real question is, How much are you willing to say yes to yourself?

Most of us have no problem saying yes to other people; as women, we are experts at giving and nurturing and doing for others. But to live a boldly beautiful life, we can't give only to others and not to ourselves. We can't cut ourselves off from all that is good and desirable and exciting and fun in the world.

We need to learn to be just as good at receiving as we are at giving. So today, our thirty-sixth day together, I encourage you to open your arms. Remember, you are a benevolent child of the universe, and everything that you desire is out there and waiting for you. It's your divine right to have it all, to be it all, and to do it all. All you need to do is open your arms and your eyes and your heart and say yes.

Today is your day. Just do it.

Just say yes.

WHAT REALLY WORKS FOR ME

It takes courage to say yes. It takes courage to accept that you actually deserve all that your heart desires—because it expands your world and your boundaries. What worked for me was finding that courage. I stood up and accepted the fact that I truly deserve what I want from life, and that I am not going to settle for less, period. As for the details of "how," I leave those to the universe.

Basically, I would advise you to define your "what" (the thing you want from the universe), say yes to it, and surrender the "how." You deserve it!

Day 37:
I HIDE MY DARK SIDE.
I EMBRACE MY DARK SIDE.

Dwell not on the past. Use it to illustrate a point, then leave it behind. Nothing really matters except what you do now in this instant of time. From this moment onward, you can be an entirely different person, filled with love and understanding, ready with an outstretched hand, uplifted and positive in every thought and deed.
— Eileen Caddy, *God Spoke to Me*

Welcome to Day 37. For the past week, we've talked about different things we can do to live our most beautiful lives—ways to create beauty all around us and approach the world and the people around us from a place of strength and openness and joy.

But what about the parts of us that aren't exactly joyful?

We've already talked a little about dealing with negative emotions, and that was a great first step. But today I want to go a little further and talk about the places inside us that just don't want to conform to this new idea of inner beauty and this new way of approaching life, no matter how many deep breaths we take or minutes we spend thinking beautiful thoughts.

No matter how hard we try or how hard we work to get rid of it, we all have darkness inside of us.

The question is, Are you able to dance with your darkness?

Can you look it in the eye and accept it, and even value it for what it is?

Or does the very fact that you have a dark side frighten you, or make you want to hide or stifle the not-so-perfect parts of yourself?

I want to be honest with you. I am not always all about beauty and goodness and light. I have a dark side—we all do. The fact is, none of us are perfect, nor should we expect ourselves to be. Our mental and spiritual flaws, like our physical flaws, are what make us human. They're what make us real. And they are just as valid a part of us as the parts that are filled with beauty and light.

As we become more enlightened, more empowered, and more awakened as women, we need to remember every day that we are not being asked to be perfect. We are being asked to acknowledge all aspects of ourselves and to love ourselves at a very deep level—the good, the bad, and the ugly. There really is no bad or ugly, no matter how negative those dark parts of us are. They add spice, they add depth, they add a little something extra to who we are. And although it is definitely advisable to control our darkness and try not to give in to it, it is just as advisable to accept that there will be days when we do.

Our darkness makes us human. And do you know what? It also makes us beautiful.

As human beings, we are constantly learning. We are here on this planet to learn and to grow—our souls require it to be fulfilled and be at their best. In a universe where learning is the primary objective, there can be no mistakes. Remember that from the first part of our journey?

Often what we perceive as a mistake is really just a lesson, designed to teach us something or help us grow in some way.

Well, there are lessons to be learned in our darkness. Lessons about jealousy and anger. Lessons about bitterness and fear. Whatever form our darkness takes, it comes from a real place inside of us that was hurt in some way. If we are really to learn and to grow, we have to embrace that aspect of ourselves and dance with it.

The really beautiful thing is that on the other side of our darkness is our light. If we want to shine our light on the world and be these wonderful light beams illuminating everyone and everything we know, we also have to acknowledge that there's something at the other end of the spectrum. Our darkness is just as real and just as valid, so we shouldn't be afraid of it, or hide it, or feel bad about ourselves because of it.

Our darkness is part of who we are, of all that exists within us. To the degree that we can dance with that aspect of ourselves and openly accept that part of ourselves, we will free ourselves to be even more filled with light, more filled with love and gratitude and respect for ourselves.

Remember, your darkness is a part of you. It makes you who you are. It makes you beautiful.

WHAT REALLY WORKED FOR ME

It was always difficult for me to get past that feeling that I had to be perfect ... *all* the time. After all, if I'm supposed to be an expert on inner beauty, how can I, of all people, let anyone see my ugly side? But as I worked and got in touch with my soul, I realized that all of us have this dark side, and that it is a real and important part of me.

Of course, to embrace my darkness, I had to find places where it was safe to let her out. I started to surround myself with people who truly accepted all of me, the light and the dark. On those days when I felt down or confused or uncertain, I reached out to those people and asked for help, support, or clarity. I learned to stop trying to do it all by myself and do it perfectly. I accepted *all* aspects of myself and accepted reality, and have achieved a new level of excellence instead.

Day 38:
I DESERVE NOTHING.
I DESERVE EVERYTHING!

Set your sights high, the higher, the better. Expect the most wonderful things to happen, not in the future but right now. Realise that nothing is too good. Allow absolutely nothing to hamper you or hold you up in any way.
— Eileen Caddy, *Footprints on the Path*

As we get closer and closer to the end of our time together, ideally you are feeling more beautiful than ever before, inside and out. I hope you've discovered a core of strength and peace you never knew you had. You might feel like, as a New 10, you are ready to conquer the world.

Well, guess what? That's what today is all about.

Today I want to focus on a very important aspect of living a more powerful, more aware, and more beautiful life as a woman. I want to talk about developing what is called a prosperity consciousness. That basically means directing your thinking in a way that enables the things you want to come to you.

Some of us don't feel entirely comfortable talking, or even thinking, about prosperity. Maybe we feel that it's greedy to want or ask for things.

Or maybe we feel like certain things we want or dream of are simply beyond our reach, so we shouldn't even let ourselves think about them.

Well, I want to take today to tell you that you it's okay to want things. In fact, it's your divine right as a woman, and as a human being.

The best part is that when you want things, when you reach for things, you open the door and allow them to come to you.

It is important to understand that you really are entitled to have the things that you most want from life. Prosperity is your birthright as a woman and as a human being. The universe has everything you could ever want, all available to you right now. The scary thing is, you could actually be stopping yourself from getting those things without even knowing it.

More often than not, we are the only thing standing between ourselves and the prosperity we so desperately want and richly deserve. We tell ourselves that what we want is impossible, or beyond our grasp, or that we don't deserve it. And guess what happens? We immediately send a message to the universe that we should not have that particular thing. No matter how much we want it and how much we deserve it, we won't get it. Because the universe listens.

The key is to become aware that your source of happiness, of health, of income, of anything at all that you desire is God—or the universe, or however you see the divine power that guides us. We need to learn to trust in that power and trust that it will deliver what is right for us if we only ask.

We also need to understand that although that divine power is ultimately our source for everything, the channels to receiving what we most desire can show up in many different forms, and in many different ways.

Including some pretty surprising ways.

Personally, I love surprises. I've come to understand a little about how the universe works, and when I desire something, when I set the intention to allow God to bring it to me, I actually ask that it come to me through surprising channels. By saying right up front that I expect to be surprised, I tell my subconscious to let go and get on with life and not obsess about how or when it's going to happen. I let it happen however it is supposed to happen.

I've actually discovered that part of the fun is standing back and watching the effortless way things unfold in my life when I allow the universe to provide for me. I anticipate how things will unfold, but I don't try to control them. I know that prosperity is mine for the asking. All I have to do is lay the groundwork and then let it happen.

Developing your own prosperity consciousness can be fun and mysterious and surprising for you too. All you need to do is remember that you are worth it, that you deserve it, and that you can and *will* have the things you need and want. Just ask the universe for them, and then let go. They will come to you.

Because you know what? You're worthy of all your dreams and goals and desires. When you tell the universe what you desire and want, and you're not sending out negative messages that you don't really deserve it, you can trust the universe to provide it. You have the power to make prosperity happen.

That's the kind of power that comes with living a boldly beautiful life.

WHAT REALLY WORKED FOR ME

Yes, I will admit it here. My name is Dawn and I am a control freak. Or at least, I was. We'll get to this in more detail in the next chapter, but I felt that if good things were going to happen to me, I had to *make* them happen. I have since learned that living in harmony with the universe means letting go and *letting* things happen.

It doesn't mean not trying and it doesn't mean not believing. It means trusting in the goodness and unlimited bounty of the universe, and realizing that the universe would give me everything I wanted and needed if I allowed it. On the other hand, if I doubted the universe, all that negative energy would drive those very things I wanted away.

Again, this is an area where I am far from perfect, especially when I "know intuitively" that I am on the threshold of a surprising, yet very earned, breakthrough Just ask my friends at 12listen and 12angel ☺! Maybe expectations and excitement aren't so easy to banish. But I think the key is to let go of the negative things like fears and doubts surrounding your desires. Instead, just trust and allow.

Day 39:
I MAKE THINGS HAPPEN.
I LET THINGS HAPPEN.

Every moment of your life is infinitely creative and the Universe is endlessly bountiful. Just put forth a clear enough request, and everything your heart desires must come to you.
— Shakti Gawain, *Creative Visualization*

Hello again. Welcome to Day 39—only one more day to go on our journey after today. I can't believe our time together is almost over. But I feel really confident that you've gained a lot from our experiences. I know in my heart that you are already living as a New 10, shining your beauty on everyone and everything you see, and ideally getting the most out of your beautiful life.

At this point, we're looking past our own beauty to the things that are necessary to living that kind of really beautiful, blessed life. Today I want to talk about a huge aspect of that. I want to talk to you about the art of surrender.

We talked a little about this whole concept yesterday when we were looking at prosperity. It's important for us to learn how to surrender our goals and our dreams and our desires to the universe. The reason is that this allows the universe to bring to us everything that we want with divine timing and through divine channels.

I hope that by now you understand that what you ask for is never wrong. It is perfectly right to ask for what you want.

The problem most of us have is that we want to control everything. We try to stipulate particular outcomes, or we have our mind set on an outcome happening at a specific time or in a specific way. What we should be doing is trusting that the universe knows what's best for us, and that what we need and want and desire will come to us in the right way at the right time.

When we try too hard to control what happens, we wind up inhibiting the universe and getting in the way. We block the universe from bringing us what we need for our highest good when we try to unlock the mystery of how it works and control what happens.

This is a natural and normal thing. A lot of us like to know everything in advance; it's just how some of us are wired. We want to know exactly what is coming, and when, and how. We like to plan and prepare so we'll be ready for anything. We'll be ready for disaster. We'll be ready for disappointment.

Unfortunately, when we get ready for disaster and disappointment, that's exactly what we invite into our lives.

So understand right now that you can't control the universe. You can certainly influence it with your thoughts—which is why negative thoughts can be so dangerous. That's also why it is so much better not to try to control outcomes, but to simply surrender.

The Law of Visualization is very clear about this. All we need to do is get clear on what we want, on what we desire, and visualize it as if we already have it. We need to know we deserve it and that it is coming. Then, once we set very clear intentions about receiving what we want and desire, we need to let go and trust in God or the universe to bring them to us.

We don't always know what form these things will take when they arrive. Oftentimes, the universe knows better than we do and brings us things in a higher form than we anticipated. Sometimes, we might not know what that higher form is; we might not even recognize it.

When we practice surrender, we are able to receive what we have asked for in that higher form. We are open and ready to accept what we most desire in its highest form of expression, even if that isn't how we pictured or imagined it.

When we surrender to the universe and simply let good and beautiful things come to us, what we create is lasting, loving, and full of light. It fulfills its divine purpose and it's done on divine timing, which makes it a win/win situation for everybody.

I encourage you to state your intentions. Set your goals. Ask for what you want and trust that you deserve it, and you can and will receive it. Then, at that moment, learn the art of surrender. Have faith in the universe. Trust in God.

Your beautiful life will come to you, in the most beautiful way possible.

WHAT REALLY WORKS FOR ME

I learned and rely on a process called "active faith." What this means is that when I desire something, I go through a very specific process. First, I make a clear decision about what it is that I desire. Once I know what that thing is, I visualize it. I then set clear intentions and I pray, asking for "this or something better."

Then—and this is the tricky part!—I let go. I surrender the outcome, the timing, and the details to the universe, and I move on with my life.

By surrendering and trusting, instead of worrying and dwelling, I open myself to the guidance I need to take appropriate action, so that when the thing I desire actually comes to me, I will recognize it and do what it takes to bring it into my life.

Faith, Trust, Surrender, and Action. ... Try it. It really works!

Day 40:
I AM IMPATIENT.
I AM PATIENT.

No pressure, no diamonds.
Mary Case—

This is it. It's Day 40 of our New 10 beauty campaign and our very last day together. I sincerely hope I have inspired you to transform yourself into the "10" that you really are, and to uncover the unique, amazing beauty that lies deep inside you. I hope that you will know, from today onward, that you are intrinsically, divinely beautiful. I hope you have learned to completely embrace yourself for who you are and to shine your light brightly in the world.

Today the last thing I'd like to discuss with you is the concept of patience. Patience is something we all need at one time or another—yet for some reason it's something we all struggle with from time to time. Remember when you were a little girl and just couldn't wait to open your Christmas presents? A lot of us are still like that now, as adults. We're never more impatient than at times when we're waiting for things to change. Whether we're dieting, trying to make more money, or looking for the right relationship, we want it all to happen *right now*! But part of the beauty of life is sitting back and letting it unfold. If all we get is the destination, we miss the journey. And sometimes, the journey really is the best part.

That's why patience can be so magical and powerful. When we finally let go and just allow things to just unfold naturally, we are able to live fully in the present moment instead of putting all our energies into that future thing that we're waiting for. We're able to enjoy every moment of every single day, since we're not viewing it as just another obstacle standing between us and our goals.

You may have noticed that patience is a lot like surrendering. In fact, it is a very specific kind of surrender. It's surrendering to the present moment, to our present reality, and trusting that whatever we're waiting for will come, that things will work out. And enjoying the gift that we have *right now*, which is today, this moment, this space, this time.

As we grow older, time moves really quickly. If we spend all our time rushing toward the things we want, we can actually forget to enjoy the now. If we're waiting to go out and enjoy our life until we lose twenty pounds or get a better job, think of every day we're wasting that we could be enjoying. If we decide we can't be happy until we find the right man, we waste every day we could be enjoying and celebrating and living our lives until that happens.

Honestly, life moves fast. So wherever you are right now, be patient that what you have asked for will come. And enjoy the gift of now.

Of course you've heard the saying "Patience is a virtue." You've probably heard it hundreds of times. But have you ever really thought about it? Patience is definitely a virtue, but it isn't a virtue just because it "improves you" or makes you a "better person" than you were before. Yes, it makes you a better parent, and partner, and friend. But the main reason patience is a virtue is because of what it does *for you*. It helps you enjoy every moment and actually lets you live a better life, a life filled with joy and free from stress.

Like most things that help you live a better life, patience makes you more beautiful. When you are patient, when you aren't stressing out waiting and wondering when things will happen, you aren't trying to force things and you are living in the moment. Your life flows smoothly and magically and effortlessly. You are filled with serenity and grace.

Today, on our last day together, I want you to think about the gift of patience, and about giving this priceless gift to yourself. Of course, if you aren't patient all the time, that's okay too, because the main person you need to be patient with in this world is yourself.

Give yourself space to grow, time to learn, and room to bloom.

Your beauty will grow every day, both inside and outside.

That's really what being a New 10 is all about. But of course you know that. Because a New 10 is exactly what you are.

WHAT REALLY WORKS FOR ME

I have shared many of the thoughts, mind-sets, meditations, and courses that have worked for me to become a New 10 woman. Although I know I am not perfect, I am honored to be able to tell you what has worked for me on my journey to recognize and celebrate the New 10 that I am.

Remember, I didn't get this way overnight. Sometimes waiting for changes to take effect can be the hardest part—and that's where patience comes in. However, although I am definitely still learning in this regard, I can honestly say that I have learned to become much more patient and I have learned and grown …

… but I am still a New 10 woman in progress, with you and for you.

That is what is so infinitely beautiful and perfect—just "being" in the process of becoming all that we are capable of, and enjoying the process as thoroughly as we can each and every day. That's part of what patience is all about: fully enjoying what is, instead of focusing on what is to be. And when you look at it that way, patience really isn't that difficult at all.

So be patient. Do you know how beautiful you are? I do.

CONCLUSION

That's it. Our forty days together are up. I hope you have enjoyed the experience and gotten to know that amazing, beautiful creature called "you" a little better. I hope you've learned to honor her feelings, to forgive her faults, and to celebrate her many, many strengths. You are a beautiful woman—a New 10 woman—and just by being here, you make the world a brighter, more beautiful place.

Before I go, I want to thank you for being a part of this campaign. My goal is for the New 10 movement to become a worldwide movement that empowers and inspires women everywhere to be everything they are meant to be. I want to see women from all walks of life learning to be strong and free and joyful and beautiful. I want each and every one of us to truly feel that love and divine beauty within. And I want us to honor our spirits and our souls and express our beauty boldly—in other words, to live a boldly beautiful life.

We are all on this earth to live the best lives we can and to take advantage of everything the universe offers us. Let me wish you all the blessings, all the luck, all the magic, all the beauty that exists in the world to help you on your journey to living a really big, really beautiful, really bold life.

Remember the New 10 Beauty Quotient Quiz I had you take before we started? You will see it again on the following page. I invite you to take it again, just to see how far you've come over the past few weeks.

I also invite you to visit my Web site at www.thenew10.com. It's a wonderful place to meet other like-minded women. You can blog about your own New 10 experiences, and you can also schedule an appointment with me for a one-on-one assessment of your quiz or any other issues you may be experiencing on your journey.

I hope this book has touched your life as much as writing it has touched mine.

Until next time, have a very beautiful day, every day.

Blessings,
Dawn

THE NEW 10 BEAUTY QUOTIENT QUIZ

Now take this quiz again and see if your answers have changed.

PART ONE: I THINK WITH MY BEAUTIFUL MIND

1. When faced with fear, do you avoid the situation or do you allow yourself to feel it and move through it?
2. When faced with a situation where your integrity and values are in question, do you speak your truth or do you stay silent, thinking that it is easier to do so?
3. On a scale of one to ten how open-minded are you in most situations?
4. When you make a mistake or unintentionally hurt another, do you forgive yourself easily or do you harbor feelings of guilt?
5. When faced with negative emotions, are you able to express them lovingly or do you lose control or even keep them hidden inside?
6. When faced with problems, do you allow worry to take over or do you approach them with a healthy concern?
7. How well on a scale of one to ten do you honor your feelings, even if it means possible rejection from someone else?

8. On a scale of one to ten, how confident are you in who you are and your unique contribution to humanity?

9. Do you live in your comfort zone or do you allow expansion of your comfort zones on a regular basis as part of your overall evolution and growth?

10. Do you practice harmlessness at all times, or do you find it necessary to get even or get back at someone, even if only occasionally?

PART TWO: I LOVE MY BEAUTIFUL BODY

1. Do you honor the guidance of your body at all times, or do you ignore its promptings to exercise, to eat certain foods or not, and to get rest when needed?

2. Do you take the time daily to affirm that your health is perfect, regardless of appearances? Do you place your focus on health?

3. Are you energetically alive? Do your soul and spirit have the chance to shine through your body and express itself?

4. Do you breathe deeply, in a focused way, with the intention of increasing your vital life force three times a day?

5. Do you dance like no one is watching?

6. Do you work at maintaining your physical strength through exercise and other activities?

7. Do you feel safe in your sexuality?

8. Do you look in the mirror and *feel beautiful?*

9. Do you flaunt the fabulous aspects of yourself at all times?

10. Do you smile when you are alone?

PART THREE: I EXPRESS MY SPIRIT BOLDLY

1. Do you believe in a benevolent universe, one that is friendly and always working with you for your highest good?
2. Are you connected with your soul? Do you know her unique qualities, favorite colors, fragrances, desires?
3. Do you believe in your innate ability to be powerful beyond measure at all times, by your simply choosing to be so?
4. Do you lead by example, living by your truth and integrity at all times?
5. Are you grateful for the gifts and blessings bestowed upon you in the present moment each day?
6. Are you comfortable with following your divine and intuitive guidance on a daily basis?
7. Do you respect that your imagination is in part your soul trying to guide you to your highest expression in this lifetime?
8. Do you embrace expansion in all areas of your life, knowing that we are constantly evolving and capable of achieving more than we think we can?
9. Do you romance yourself, light candles for yourself, play love music for yourself, date yourself?
10. Are you able to laugh at life's challenges, knowing that in doing so you are freeing your spirit to provide you with solutions to what are actually lessons we are very capable of learning?

PART FOUR: I LIVE A BOLDLY BEAUTIFUL LIFE

1. Do you strive to become more conscious and aware of your patterns and paradigms?

2. Do you value just being, spending time with yourself and doing nothing?

3. Do you live in the present moment, or are your thoughts always focused on the past or future?

4. Do you take the time to think before you speak, especially in times of deeply felt emotions?

5. Are you willing to allow yourself to age beautifully? Are you aware that it is possible to do so?

6. Are you willing to ask for what you want from others, from yourself, and from the universe?

7. Can you dance with your darkness, knowing that she needs your love and acceptance to express and be the light?

8. Do you have a prosperity consciousness, knowing that God is your source of unlimited wealth and supply in all areas of your life, regardless of appearances to the contrary?

9. Are you able to detach from outcomes and therefore create the space for the universe to manifest with you in an easy and graceful manner?

10. Are you patient? Can you let go and trust and have faith in the divine timing of all things that are meant to be for your highest good?

FREE BONUS GIFT

Boldly Beautiful Radio at its finest.

Log on to <http://www.thenew10.com/bookbonus> and receive the three best interviews with Dawn and her guests discussing inner beauty and how to express it boldly in the world. These interviews will shed additional light as to how easy it is and why it so important to be true to yourself, to see the best in yourself and to love yourself, no matter what.

I hope you enjoy listening to them as much as I enjoyed creating them for you.

Wishing you a beautiful and magical journey,

Dawn

BUY A SHARE OF THE FUTURE IN YOUR COMMUNITY

These certificates make great holiday, graduation and birthday gifts that can be personalized with the recipient's name. The cost of one S.H.A.R.E. or one square foot is $54.17. The personalized certificate is suitable for framing and will state the number of shares purchased and the amount of each share, as well as the recipient's name. The home that you participate in "building" will last for many years and will continue to grow in value.

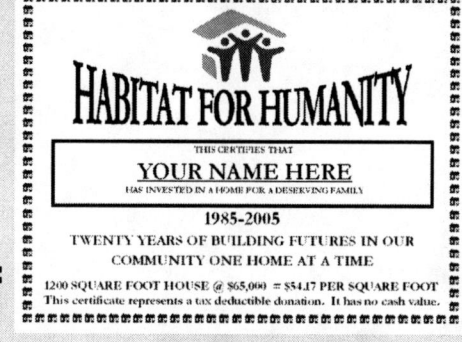

Here is a sample SHARE certificate:

Sample certificate:
HABITAT FOR HUMANITY
THIS CERTIFIES THAT
YOUR NAME HERE
HAS INVESTED IN A HOME FOR A DESERVING FAMILY
1985-2005
TWENTY YEARS OF BUILDING FUTURES IN OUR COMMUNITY ONE HOME AT A TIME
1200 SQUARE FOOT HOUSE @ $65,000 = $54.17 PER SQUARE FOOT
This certificate represents a tax deductible donation. It has no cash value.

YES, I WOULD LIKE TO HELP!

I support the work that Habitat for Humanity does and I want to be part of the excitement! As a donor, I will receive periodic updates on your construction activities but, more importantly, I know my gift will help a family in our community realize the dream of homeownership. **I would like to SHARE in your efforts against substandard housing in my community!** *(Please print below)*

PLEASE SEND ME _____ SHARES at $54.17 EACH = $ $_____

In Honor Of: _____

Occasion: (Circle One)   HOLIDAY   BIRTHDAY   ANNIVERSARY
   OTHER: _____

Address of Recipient: _____

Gift From: _____ *Donor Address:* _____

Donor Email: _____

I AM ENCLOSING A CHECK FOR $ $_____ PAYABLE TO HABITAT FOR HUMANITY <u>OR</u> PLEASE CHARGE MY VISA OR MASTERCARD *(CIRCLE ONE)*

Card Number _____ Expiration Date: _____

Name as it appears on Credit Card _____ Charge Amount $ _____

Signature _____

Billing Address _____

Telephone # Day _____ Eve _____

PLEASE NOTE: Your contribution is tax-deductible to the fullest extent allowed by law.
Habitat for Humanity • P.O. Box 1443 • Newport News, VA 23601 • 757-596-5553
www.HelpHabitatforHumanity.org